WHEN LIGHTNING STRIKES TWICE

Dear Stephanie

May lightning never strike twice in your house.

[illegible signature]

Coach's Corner

WHEN LIGHTNING STRIKES TWICE

Gina Elkon Rubin

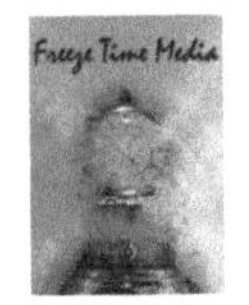

When Lightning Strikes Twice

ISBN: 978-1-946702-45-6

Freeze Time Media

Cover designer: Judy A. Tashji

To My Family and Best Friend

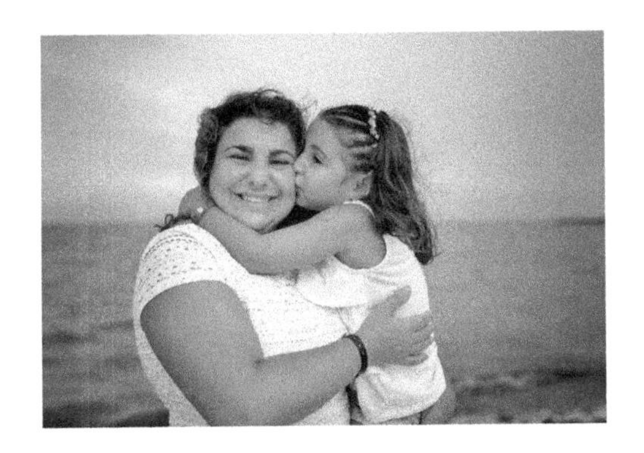

Acknowledgment

Thanks to all the individuals who helped Iliana and me through our peril. There are so many it is impossible to name them all. However, I have acknowledged some who went above and beyond on my website - www.wix.com/LightningStrikes2xs.

Even though I am lucky enough to have so many wonderful people in my life, there are a few who I will mention here. First off, my best friend and her husband, Mechal Weiss Haas and Chaim Haas. Besides being "my marketing" department for this book, Mechal and Chaim lifted mountains just to be by our side and help us in any way they could. They sent Iliana and me tons of presents (fun and emotional), called many times a day to lift our spirits, traveled many miles to see us, and did whatever was necessary to make sure we were okay. It was comforting to have them fight beside us.

My family! There are lots of them, so be patient. First my brother and his family, Ezra, Marla, Ross, and Sydnee Elkon — the saying goes, "I smile because you're my brother. I laugh because there's nothing you can do about it!" So true, but the second I need him, he is there. When he found out about Iliana, he left work and came to the hospital. Even though I inherited my sister-in-law through marriage, she acts as though we have been sisters my whole life. She, too, left work and came to the hospital as soon as she heard about Iliana. It melts my heart to know I will always have devotion by my side with them.

My nephew, Ross Elkon, spent countless hours editing this book. Prior to that when he was at the young age of 13, he wanted to shave his head, paint his nails orange, and instead of party favors for his Bar Mitzvah party, he wanted to donate the money to a cancer organization, all in honor of his little cousin. And not to be forgotten, my niece. When she heard about editing the book, she wanted in on the action.

My in-laws, Ron and Mindy Rubin, have always made themselves available to us, definitely products of their terrific upbringing. I think that because when their families heard about Iliana and me, they also did whatever they could (and still do) to help us.

With a tremendous amount of luck and thanks to God, I was born to Michael and Joan Elkon. I remember during my childhood there were times I would wish they were cooler or like someone else's parents; however, I know now how lucky I was and am. Even if we disagree, my parents have always supported me in my endeavors and were always around when I needed someone to turn to. I take their love for granted because I am fortunate it will always cloak me.

And last but certainly not least, my husband and kids. My husband, Josh, had a tremendous amount to endure. Besides having to be the breadwinner, he cured Sarah and Ithan's boo-boos, chauffeured all of us around, cuddled Iliana when she was scared or needed love, and still found time to nurse me back to health, physically and emotionally. Somehow through all that, he still made us laugh.

Sarah, my oldest, tried not to cause Josh or me any grief as she knew we had so much to handle already. As soon as she heard about Iliana she jumped into action, fundraising in different ways. In fact, due to her efforts with the Leukemia & Lymphoma Society, she has raised over $70,000 for them.

Ithan, my middle child and only son, inherited Josh's humor and my big smile. In fact, he caused Iliana and me to laugh through our whole awful journey with cancer.

My youngest, my MVP, Iliana. Even though she is still a child, she has had to endure more than most people do in a lifetime. Her love of life and persistence to always survive is a lesson to us all. Without her constant smile and humor, I am not sure how I would have endured my diagnosis.

Contents

Preface **xiii**
Iliana's Igloo **xv**
Vacation 1
What's Wrong with Iliana? 7
Leukemia 15
Reactions 23
First Days in the Hospital 27
Accessing the Port — Sara Willis 33
Two Kids —Their Desire to Help 39
Pancreatitis 49
School Starts — Not for Everyone 59
My Daughter Saved My Life **63**
When Lightning Strikes Twice 65
Confirmation 71
Our Mayberry 79
Don't Fear Striking Out — Play the Game 83
My Nephew's Moment to Shine 87
Benefit at Coach's Corner 93
Chemotoxicity 101
Iliana is Back at School 109
Girls Can Fight **121**
We are Done! 123
Thunder Keeps Rolling: Life After Cancer **129**
Cancer Keeps on Giving 131
Team LoCo on Cancer 135
No Confidence 139
Testimony 143

Preface

I can still remember every second, every moment, of that fateful day. I can still remember every sight, every detail, of Fairfax Hospital. I can still remember every thought, every emotion in that small piece of time. The fear when the doctor sat my husband and me down, took a deep breath, and with sorrow in his eyes, said those four words, those six life-changing, earth-shattering syllables: "Your daughter has cancer."

My name is Gina Rubin. My husband's name is Josh, and we have three children: Sarah, Ithan and Iliana. On July 22, 2015, we were told that Iliana, my youngest daughter, age six, had acute lymphoblastic leukemia. The news shocked our family, our friends, and our community; it was a true lightning strike to our hearts. The storm that arose encapsulated us all, but this was a thunderstorm, and then lightning struck twice.

About six weeks after Iliana's initial diagnosis, I was diagnosed with Burkitt lymphoma, another form of blood cancer. I was shocked that two out of five members of my generally healthy family had been diagnosed with cancer. A mother and daughter diagnosed with blood cancer at the same time is almost unheard of. This is a story that needs to be heard, so here is our story.

Part One

Iliana’s Igloo

1

Vacation

My name is Gina Rubin. I am happily married to my husband, Josh, and we have three wonderful children: Sarah, Ithan, and Iliana. We live in a beautiful community filled with extraordinary people in Purcellville, Virginia, only twenty minutes from both my parents and my in-laws. My brother, Ezra, and his wife, Marla, don't live much further away, with my nephew and niece, Ross and Sydnee. I am lucky to have many close friends that live both near and far. Without the support of all of these people, I wouldn't have been able to weather the storm of the next few years.

Our ordeal began in the summer of 2015. The kids were excited to get out of school and I was excited to spend some quality time with the family. Our summer was filled to the brim with plans: camps, relaxation, and to top it all off, one big vacation for all of us. We were going to California for the wedding of a family friend, and while we were there, planned to take the kids to nearby Disneyland. We were going on the trip with my in-laws, Ron and Mindy Rubin, known by my kids as

Zeidie and Bubbie, and whom I adore. On July 9, 2015, we set off on our vacation. The plane ride to San Francisco was Iliana's first flight, and afterward, we drove to Anaheim. We arrived a few days prior to the wedding to allow for us to enjoy ourselves. While in San Jose, we visited nearby San Francisco and did the typical tourist things, including going to Ghirardelli Square. In order to get to Ghirardelli Square, we had to walk up a steep hill. Iliana complained her legs hurt, so much so that she refused to walk up to the Ghirardelli store. In hindsight, I should have noticed something off with my typically sweets-loving daughter, but at the time, I thought she was just being a diva. I sat with her while everyone else got ice cream and, though I now regret it, chastised her for refusing to walk.

After exploring San Francisco for a while, we went to the wedding, which was phenomenal.

The wedding was beautiful, and the ceremony was touching. At the reception, there happened to be a photo booth. Iliana was in pretty much every picture. She dressed up with props, ran back and forth from the photo booth to our table, and provided us with many laughs. She seemed to have been back to normal, which only furthered the idea that she had been a diva earlier.

After the excitement of the wedding, we drove to Anaheim on the Pacific Coast Highway. This is a very scenic route, complete with beautiful mountain vistas and outstanding views. At one stop, we saw sea lions. Most of us got out of the car to see them, but Iliana was too tired to walk with us.

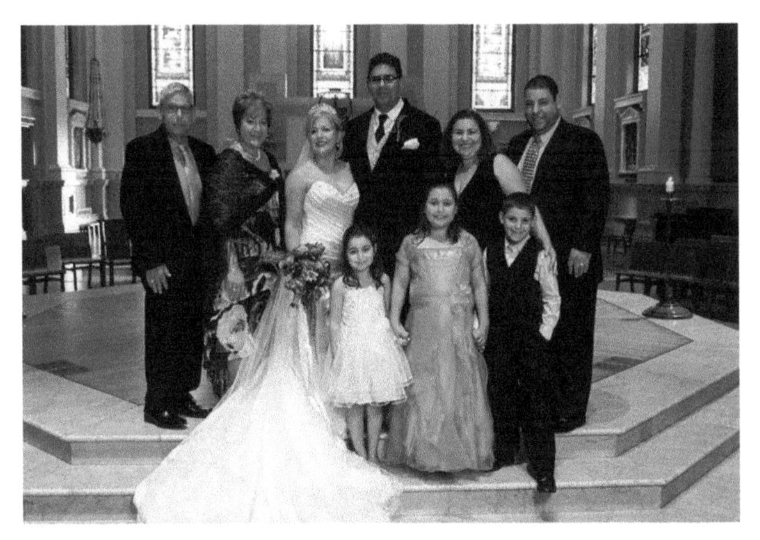

Ron, Mindy, Lisa, Jose and us at Lisa and Jose's wedding.

We met up with my cousin, Kim, whom I had not seen for over thirty years. The kindness with which she and her husband, Brad, welcomed us into their home would have made one think that we had seen them just the other day.

She invited us for dinner, to which we were late. Typically, this would be caused by our poor time management skills, known amongst our family and friends as Rubin Standard Time, or RST. This particular instance was not our fault, for our rental car had broken down. Once we finally arrived at their house, we had a wonderful evening.

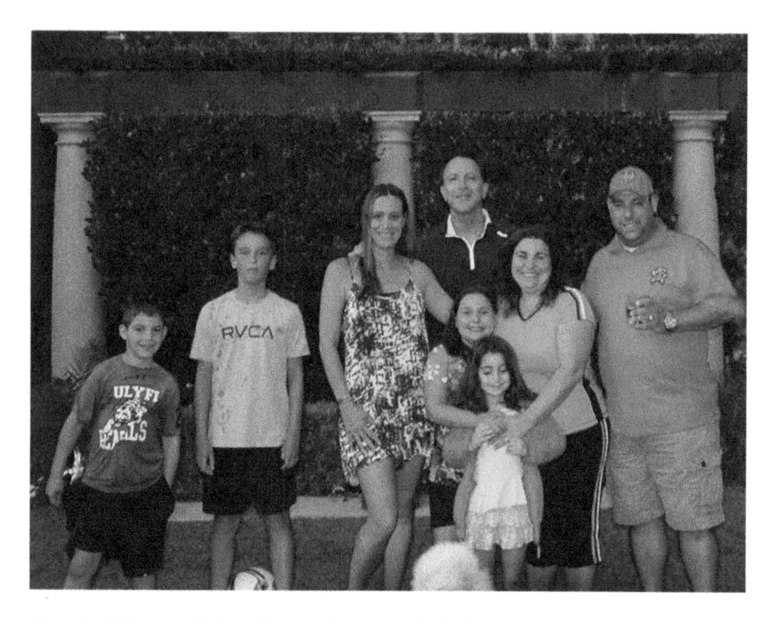

Brad, Kim and family and us at their home in North Beach.

We got to Anaheim and settled in the house we had reserved for a few days. It had great amenities, including a pool and a stroller. On our first day there, we went to California Adventure, another Disney park adjacent to Disneyland. We ended up taking the stroller with us to the park in case Iliana had more leg pain. The park was very fun; we spent the whole day there, in which we rode all the rides and had a blast. Iliana stayed in the stroller and once again, I thought she was just being a diva. She seemed content in the stroller, so I was also happy. Josh wanted to ride the Tower of Terror, which was going to close soon, but we were in another area of the park. Iliana, the daredevil she is, wanted to go with him. In order to make it on time, he hoisted her up on his shoulders and ran to the ride. From what I heard afterward, they made it and had a blast. The next day, we went to the beach, but the water was too cold, and so we didn't go in.

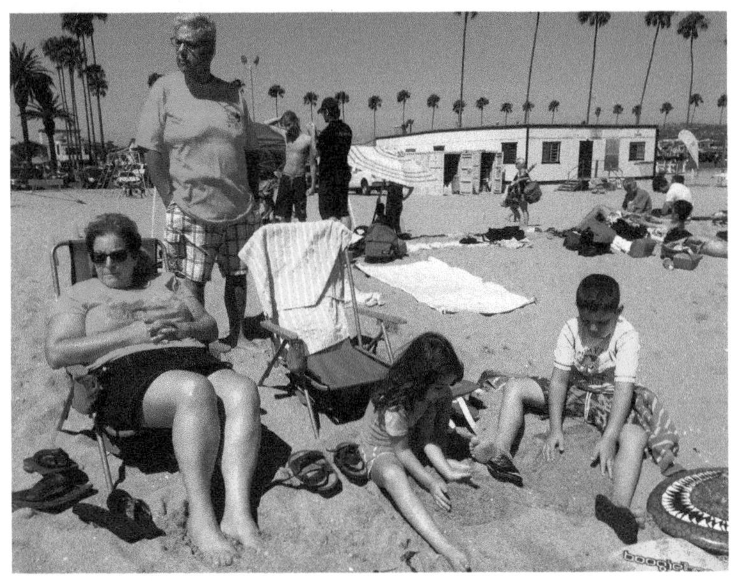

Ron, Mindy, Ithan and Iliana at the beach.

While in Anaheim, our dear friend, Racquel Russell, surprised the kids and joined us. With her, we enjoyed a lot of the tourist locations, including Roscoe's Chicken and Waffles. On Friday, we finally went to Disneyland, where I once again brought the stroller. It was Disney's one-hundredth anniversary, which was celebrated with cupcakes. We rode It's A Small World, Thunder Mountain, and all of the other Disneyland attractions.

Most of us went back to the house for a few hours, but Josh and Ithan decided to stay at the park to get Ithan over his fear of upside-down roller coasters. It worked, and in fact, if Ithan doesn't go on to be a Major League Baseball player, he wants to be a roller coaster designer.

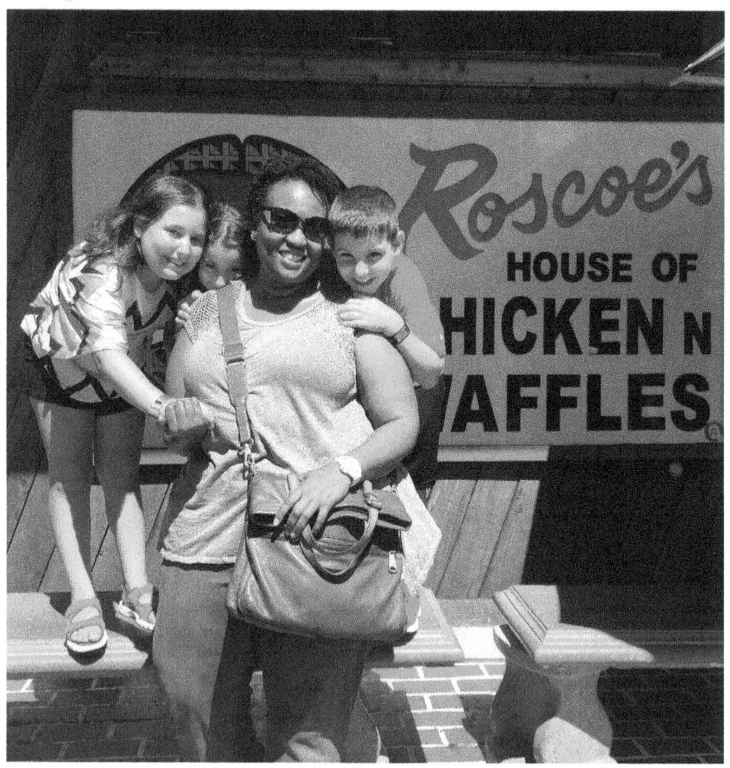

Racquel and the kids.

2

What's Wrong with Iliana?

We got home from our trip on July 19, 2015, and Iliana went to the doctor the next day. Her leg pain had gotten to an unbearable point, she became exceedingly fatigued, and we noticed that she looked extremely pale. In hindsight, she was pale the entire trip, and it is very apparent in our vacation photos. Josh took her to Loudoun Pediatrics, a nearby pediatric center that has walk-in capabilities. The doctor needed to take Iliana's blood, and after a bit of calming and convincing, we got her to allow the doctor to take her blood. The doctor put in a rush order for blood tests so that they would arrive back the same day, rather than the several day wait time. I suspect the doctor had an idea about her ailment, but, without confirmation, didn't say anything.

Josh was with Ithan at a baseball assessment when the doctor called him that evening. She told him Iliana's blood counts were very low and she was anemic. He needed to take Iliana to the pediatric emergency room at Fairfax Hospital immediately. We have a much closer hospital, but at the time, the pediatric ER in Fairfax was more well-versed to handle Iliana's condition. Josh left immediately to get Iliana and me from the house. Ithan got a ride home with our good friend, Adam Sanborn. His wife, Meghan, emailed me later that night mentioning that it was "*Very scary when Josh rushed out of tryouts...*" I was making dinner when Josh walked in, and I left in such a rush that I left dinner out.

I called my neighbor and close friend, Cathy Fain, to watch Sarah and Ithan while we were gone. Luckily, my parents, Joan and Michael Elkon (Oma and Zeida to my kids), live only 20 minutes away. Cathy watched Sarah and Ithan until my mother came over. I have no idea what was going through their young minds, but I can only imagine their fear and terror at the situation. It was probably difficult and confusing for them to not know what was going on. Josh quickly drove to the ER. Josh is the Mario Andretti of our area, so quickly means as fast as the car would go. I believe I heard later that the Loudoun County Sheriff's Office was still trying to identify that UFO. Little did we know we would have to drive this route many times in the coming months.

When we got to the ER, we had the car valet parked. The INOVA hospital system understands that when you have to run to the ER, the last thing you want to think about is your car. I have heard that you do not want to "not" wait at the ER if others are already there, but it is true. Without a doubt, it is hard to be at the ER and see a loved one suffer, but trust me, you want to wait. I say that because as soon as we told the ER staff who we were, we were told that the pediatrician had called ahead and we were taken back immediately.

Once again, Iliana's blood had to be taken. Once again, to say the least, she was not happy about it. She thrashed and cried, but the vampires, sorry, phlebotomists, finally got her blood. It is so hard to see your child, at any age, be in pain and not really be able to do anything. I was devastated and I wanted to take all of the pain she was feeling into myself. All I really wanted was for the doctor to tell me nothing was wrong and that I could take Iliana home.

Unfortunately, that did not happen. Waiting for the blood results was torture. My husband was strong, but I had to excuse myself to go to the bathroom to cry. I didn't want to cry in front of Iliana because I didn't want her to know her parents were scared. In the bathroom, my imagination got the best of me. What is wrong with her? Would she be okay? When could we go home? When will I wake up from this nightmare? What if she had cancer?

My thoughts created such turmoil in my head; little did I know the horrible answer. I finally managed to compose myself and went back to her room in the ER. Josh and I tried to make jokes and laugh to lighten the mood, but we were scared. I was terrified of the uncertainty, even though knowing would mean our fears could come true. The nurses kept coming in to make sure we were okay. I was unaware they feared the worst. Finally, the doctor came in with a smile and said that Iliana did not have cancer. I let out a sigh of relief. I was so thankful, thinking my fear of her getting cancer wasn't realized. I was not aware that the test he was referring to only covered easily detectable cancers, late-stage cancers, or tumors.

I did not know that the initial screening did not include blood cancer. The nurses and doctor in the ER couldn't figure out why her blood counts were so low. We were told to stay overnight and we were put in a room in the oncology and hematology ward. I didn't know that meant the medical field in Fairfax still knew something wasn't right and that it takes a few days for blood to be evaluated in many different ways.

Josh decided to stay with Iliana and I went home to relieve my mom and to be with the other kids. I was being optimistic, thinking that Iliana was fine and that she did not have cancer. Maybe she was just sick, or she just ate some bad seafood in California.

In the back of my head, I was still worried. Even though I got home late, the kids were still up. Both my mother and my kids had a lot of questions, most of which I could not answer. The only things I knew for sure were that we still had no clue why Iliana's blood counts were low and that we were going back to the hospital in the morning. The kids slept with me, mostly because they were scared, but I also needed to have them close.

It must have been quite the funny scene. On my bed were our two chocolate labrador retrievers, Baxter, who is at least eighty pounds and stretches to about five feet, and Annie, who was about sixty pounds; Sarah; Ithan and myself. That night, I slept fitfully. It was hard to sleep as many terrifying thoughts danced through my head, taunting my optimism, taunting me. The next morning, I drove to Fairfax Hospital with Sarah and Ithan in tow. Iliana was hooked up to machines, but in my mind, that was standard for hospitals. I was trying to be positive, not just for the kids, but for myself as well. The hospital was doing tests on Iliana's blood.

My parents and in-laws came to the hospital as well. You would have thought that we were having a party when, in actuality, we were all very worried because we did not know what was going on with Iliana. At one point, I looked around and could not find my father-in-law. I found him in a doorway, far from everyone else, crying. He looked at me and said, with a pleading, sorrowful look in his eyes, "*I want my granddaughter to be okay*." He had verbalized all of our greatest fears in seven heartbreaking words. With as much courage as I could muster, I tried to reassure him that everything would be okay. Funny how I could be strong for him, but not for myself.

Our friends, who are our kids' "adopted grandparents," Roger and Toni Hampton, also known as Pops and Nona, came when they heard we were in the hospital. I've recently asked Toni how she felt when she saw us, and she said, "*When Roger and I first came to the hospital, I think it was a Tuesday, Josh fell into my arms and cried. I glanced over and saw you, and I'll never forget the look on your face. It was like you had the whole world in your arms and didn't know what to do. This may sound silly yet these were my thoughts. I'll never forget it. At that moment I decided I needed to help you — in any way I could. My mind was racing, how I could do this and what you would need and it came down to the simplest thing — I'll take care of your house. You all would need clean underwear and sheets. I think I told you that day I would help you. Yet I don't really remember that part.*"

My brother, Ezra, and his wife, Marla, came to the hospital as soon as they could. They immediately left work to come to see us when they heard what was going on. Ezra had been an EMT for over fifteen years, but at the time was working for the Capitol Police as a hazmat specialist, and had also been a paramedic for a few years. Marla holds a bachelor's degree in radiologic sciences. In that way, they both held a background in the medical field. Based on the information that we had given them, they both had already feared that Iliana had leukemia.

My brother and I are very different people. I love crowds, being the center of attention, having lots of friends, and am far from shy. Ezra is happy to be in the back, enjoys having a few close-knit friends, and is quiet if he doesn't know you. Ezra took Sarah with him to get Slurpees. It gave him a chance to talk to her about what was going on with Iliana. We love Slurpees, all the sugary, cold goodness you could want. Sarah was asking him questions about leukemia, so he was honest with her. She was googling leukemia anyway, so it made more sense for someone close to her to tell her the truth. I am glad he spoke to her because I don't think that I could have explained anything to her without crying and scaring her. It was good to see him there and I'm happy he came. Even though we are so different, he has a calming effect on me.

Marla is such an amazing person. I remember when Sarah had her tonsils out, she had to go back in for surgery because a blood vessel popped. The doctor was not worried, but I was. When I saw Marla, I broke down. She stayed with me and kept me calm. The in-law part is the legal terminology, but for me, she is the sister I never had. We disagree on some things, but I know I can always count on her. After Ezra left to go take care of Ross and Sydnee, Marla stayed with us at the hospital for a few more hours.

That night, I stayed in the hospital with Iliana while Josh took the kids home. We still did not know what was going on with Iliana, but with each passing moment of not getting results, I felt reassured that we were going to be told that everything was fine. Once I was told it was not one form of cancer, I never thought it could be another form, even though we were in the pediatric oncology (cancer) ward. The waiting and not knowing was torture, but once again I thought for sure this was something that would pass, that is until after I spoke to the resident. Fairfax Hospital is a teaching hospital and everyone was wonderful, including the students. I asked the resident, a student, about Iliana and told him that the ER said it was not cancer. He gave me a weird look that shook me to my core and said that he was surprised the ER would say that, because it could be leukemia. Her blood was being examined in many different ways to see why her blood count was so low, which is why it took so long to get results. He explained to me that once her blood was checked one way, if nothing was found, it was put in a centrifuge and viewed a different way. He told us that he would speak to Doctor Schorin again, but leukemia was what Doctor Schorin had said was the most possible explanation. Doctor Marshall A. Schorin, from Pediatrics Specialists of Virginia (PSV), was one of the various doctors who checked on Iliana while she was in the hospital. PSV has a lot of doctors who come in to check on the oncology and hematology patients. I was still hoping that Iliana would be fine, that she would hop out of bed and say "Gotcha!" The nurse had to come in every few hours to check Iliana's vitals, and I would ask every time about Iliana's results. The nurse told me each time that nothing had been found yet, so yet again I believed everything was fine. My mind would not, could not, imagine another outcome.

The next morning, Josh and the kids came back to the hospital. Our friend Ryan also came with his daughter, Ashlyn. Ryan had cancer when he was nineteen and managed to make a full recovery. I wish he never experienced what it meant to be diagnosed with cancer, but it helped to know he knew what to expect regardless of Iliana's outcome. He took Sarah and Ithan home so they did not have to be in the hospital all day. Sarah recorded some of the conversation in the car, and in true Ryan style, he kept the kids laughing with his goofy stories. She played some of the conversation for me, which made me feel better. Hearing my kids laugh and sound happy gave me strength and hope. I knew they were scared but it was important to know that they were in good hands, well taken care of, and were having fun.

Meanwhile, Josh and I were in the hospital waiting to find out what was going on with Iliana. As we sat waiting, we just watched as the minutes ticked by. One second it was noon, and the next, it was midnight. It was now July 22, 2015, the day our lives changed forever.

3

Leukemia

Dr. Schorin took Josh and me into what is called the "family room" at the hospital in the oncology ward. This is where we were informed that Iliana had leukemia, specifically pre-B ALL, or acute lymphoblastic leukemia. Dr. Schorin delivered the horrific news to Josh and me in such a matter of fact tone that both of us could've mistaken him for a robot. At the time, we felt insulted that he didn't show the slightest touch of empathy, but the truth is that he could have said the same thing with puppies smothering me with kisses, and it would not have mattered. His lack of empathy was even a bit grounding for us, pulling us back to the terrible reality from the nightmares created within our minds. I felt like I had been hit by a truck. My daughter had cancer. Impossible. The stories of this happening to others had felt so distant from us, yet here we were, in one of those very stories. Dr. Schorin went on to say that he knew we did not believe him, but based on his experience, this was not the worst thing that could have happened to Iliana.

I was so dumbfounded by this news, my mind went

dark. I was numb. Iliana was so young, only six, and her world was already going to be thrown upside down. Was our house clean enough, would she see her friends, would she still have friends, would she be forced to mature and lose her innocence? What did this mean in terms of our life and what did pre-B ALL mean? I had gone through a range of emotions in just a short amount of time. First, I was scared about taking Iliana to the hospital, upset from watching her cry from the pain of the needle used to take her blood, relieved that she did not have cancer, optimistic that everything would be fine, happy about nothing in her blood having been found yet, and scared once again thanks to not knowing what was wrong with her, so that by the time we found out her diagnosis, we were numb.

Dr. Schorin asked us if we wanted a second opinion. Huh? We stared at him dumbfounded. Would it really matter? Everything said was well above our heads and even though the diagnosis was not what we wanted to hear, we just wanted Iliana to be better. A second opinion would mean traveling to a different location and waiting longer. The hardest part was having to listen to someone else who you hoped knew what he/she was talking about and not being able to even know if it was the right decision. It was not like we were going to suggest a different approach. I mean, what did we know? You truly want to believe that everything will be alright in your heart but your head is saying, "You don't know, idiot!"

The medicinal explanation for Iliana's condition is as follows. ALL is acute lymphoblastic leukemia and is defined as a tumor or cancer of the blood that starts in the bone marrow and spreads to the bloodstream. There are about 2,900 cases of ALL diagnosed in children and adolescents in the United States each year. Leukemia starts in the bone marrow and starts as a single, young white blood cell called a "blast" which develops a series of mutations that allow it to multiply uncontrollably. Eventually, blasts take over the bone marrow and crowd out normal cells. Symptoms of ALL include fatigue, paleness, fever, and bone pain (taken from Iliana's treatment handbook from INOVA Fairfax). Huh? Bored yet? Probably not if you love science; however I am not a lover of science to begin with and all I heard, like a loud megaphone blaring over and over, was "YOUR DAUGHTER HAS CANCER." It was like a pounding in my head that would not go away. Unfortunately, this was a 2.5-year headache and heartache that would always be around.

Dr. Schorin asked if we would allow Iliana to be part of a clinical trial. Treatment for her wouldn't change, but her reactions to the treatment would be officially recorded. "*Of course,*" we said, "*anything to help other sick children, as long as it doesn't affect Iliana.*" Little did we know that in the near future, Iliana would benefit from a trial.

He gave us options for her treatment, chemotherapy being the harshest but most impactful. It could cause side effects such as nausea, hair loss, mouth sores, fatigue, and other painful side effects, and some side effects were rarer than others. There were four phases of treatment: the induction phase, consolidation, delayed intensification, and maintenance.

Induction lasts for four weeks and the goal of the

phase is to kill the leukemia cells. At the end of this phase, a bone marrow aspiration, or bone marrow surgery, is done. The bone marrow is then examined under a microscope, and the hope is that the leukemia cells are gone. If so, remission begins. Even though in theory the cancer is almost eradicated, if the treatments aren't finished, the cancer has a greater possibility of coming back. The consolidation phase lasts about twelve to sixteen weeks and is a very difficult phase. The purpose of this phase is to kill any leukemia cells that weren't eradicated during the induction phase. To help accomplish this, a weekly spinal tap is done. The third phase is delayed intensification and lasts about eight weeks. This phase is done with the hopes of preventing leukemia from returning. The final phase, maintenance, can last up to three years but is less intensive than the other three phases and is the general recovery time while the body and immune system recover. Throughout all of the phases, oral and intravenous medicine is given as well as a lot of spinal taps (taken from Iliana's treatment handbook from INOVA Fairfax).

Josh drove home to get the other kids from Ryan. We decided the best thing to do was tell them at Ryan's house. He could try to help Josh answer questions the kids had, while also acting as emotional support, along with Ashlyn. I stayed in the hospital with Iliana. Inside, I was in turmoil; outside, I was crying. I didn't know how to interpret this news. My baby had cancer, and I had no idea what to think or do to help her. The whole thing made me think of a song, "Where Were You When the World Stopped Turning." I asked a number of very close family and friends what they felt when we told them about Iliana. This is what they said:

Ezra remembered, "*Soooo........ that morning you called Marla and me and told us that you were going to Fairfax Hospital with Iliana because the doctor didn't like her blood work. I remember having a sinking feeling and leaving work to come meet you at the hospital. When I got there, you hadn't seen the doctor yet. Everyone was scared but was being strong for Iliana.*

I ended up leaving before the doctor came because I had to go meet the kids when they got home from school. On my way, I was at the Battlefield Parkway exit on the Greenway when Josh called to tell me and I remember feeling it was going to be OK. I also remember telling Josh to not forget to tell the doctor that you all had stored cord blood for Iliana and that may be important at some point.

After I hung up the phone, I remember pretty much losing it all the way home. I remember us telling the kids that night and having Ross come to us at some point a few days later and saying he was ready to be part of the hair shaving party.

Marla recalled, "I was at the hospital with you and my heart sank. I felt helpless that I couldn't do anything. I wanted to fix her. I wanted to help her. I wanted to take away all of yours and Josh's pain. It wasn't fair. But I knew deep down somehow she was going to be OK. Not sure how or why, I just knew she would be fine.

Maybe it's the fighter in her, her attitude, or because you and Josh are her parents, but I knew she was going to be just fine.

When she got sick, it was almost like an out-of-body experience. Your mom was talking to me, Mindy was talking, but I can't remember anything they said. I remember thinking of Sarah and Ithan and how they were going to handle it all. I was scared for all of you."

Toni recalled thinking, "*This is unbelievable that this beautiful child has this illness. How did this happen?*"

My mom noted, "*The day after you came back from Cal, and I saw Iliana, I felt there was something seriously wrong, but wanted to stay positive.*

The next day she was admitted to Fairfax, and I called Ezra and Marla. They were concerned and didn't know what to think. "Disbelief, concern, worry, scared but at the same time hopeful for a good outcome."

I texted my best friend in the world, Mechal Weiss Haas. If I had tried to call her, she wouldn't have understood a single word through all of my crying. Mechal was the friend that was always there for me, always supporting, always holding my hand no matter what. I was extraordinarily lucky to have her. We met in a stairwell at college, and since then we have never been apart. When it comes to the best friend category, I hit the jackpot! She told me when I texted her, "*the world stopped.*"

Ithan, who was only eight, feared, "*I did not like when I heard about it. I was sad because one, I had no clue what cancer was, and two, I also didn't want it to happen again.*"

Sarah, who was ten, wrote, "*I felt like my perfect life was over. Life was so amazing and nothing was ever wrong before. I also felt like it was my fault, I felt like I had done something wrong. I also felt helpless because there was nothing I could do to change it and there was nothing I could do to make it all better.*"

I asked Josh what he felt. This was tough as I can't even comprehend what was going through his mind. Josh is a very tough cookie, but inside he is a big teddy bear with a huge heart. He is my rock, my shield, my strength, all in one package. I remember when Sarah got her tonsils out, I was okay on the outside until Josh walked in. Then, I became a blubbering fool.

He grievously remembered, "*The first thing that I thought was that my little girl was going to die. You associate cancer with death, and it tore me to the core to hear that my baby could die. What were we going to do? How were we going to live without her? Why was this happening to us? What did I do wrong that my little girl was being punished? I felt like I would have done anything in that moment to take the cancer from her and put it in my body so that she didn't have to suffer. Then it got worse. I now had to figure out how we were going to tell Sarah and Ithan. It was at that point when I realized that there was no way they were going to be able to handle the news (relatively speaking) if their father was a mess. I had to be strong, or at least give the facade that I was so that they felt comfortable, felt everything was going to be OK. But I am sure they were thinking the same things that I did when we were given that life-shattering news.*"

I had to do something, as just sitting around was making me think too much. Step one was to tell our wonderful friends. I was not sure how to put into words what was going through my mind. How does one tell the people they love, some almost like family, that your life and theirs will change forever? We were typically very social, and frequently went out and hosted parties. This would have to change.

I sent out the following email: "This is probably one of the hardest emails I hope I ever have to write. We found out a few days ago that our beautiful Iliana has leukemia. She has pre-B

ALL, which is the common form of leukemia for children. The success rate is really high, thank God, but we have a long journey ahead. Please bear with us as we will not be having people over for a while. And if you do, no one can be sick. We are going to try to keep things as normal as possible and ensure that Sarah and Ithan's lives are as amazing as possible.

We are very fortunate as we know the love that surrounds us and how wonderful our friends are. We thank God for you every day."

4

Reactions

I was told by a lot of friends how they reacted when they found out about Iliana. I believe they were more shocked than anything else; some said they had to sit down from the shock. We live in this amazing sleepy town where the most that ever happens is a cow gets loose. Hearing that a friend's child is sick is catastrophic. A lot did not know how to react or were worried they might say something stupid or insensitive.

Here are some of the emails I received:

"We can't imagine. Just know that you're in our thoughts, and if there's ANYTHING we can do...a playdate with Ithan and Sarah, a ride somewhere, errand running, casserole for dinner, etc....., please let us know."

"We will be praying for her and you guys. If there is anything we can do, we are here."

"I'm so so sorry about the terrible news!! We can't believe that you all are going through this! Thank goodness you have such a wonderful family and support system behind you. We will pray for you and for Iliana. We will be here for you in any way that you need...meals, having Sarah and Ithan over for playdates, etc."

I am lucky as my friends know that I love having fun and laughing. So even though we were bearing an unimaginable burden, my friends tried to make me laugh with funny but heartfelt emails, such as: "*Please know that we are praying for Iliana and your family and we are here to help you in any way possible. That little spitfire of yours is so fierce and feisty, I know that she will be tackling this in mad "prima-donna" style like no other girl can!!!*

Seriously, let me know what we can do - overnights, practices, yell at Ithan to do his homework, decorate Sarah's locker...anything!!! Now that I have all your family's eating requirements down, I can help out with meals too!

Please call me or pop in ANYTIME!!! I'll give you some space but I am here for you..."

"*Hey, we'd both be there to help if we could with whatever you need. Bone marrow test or transfusion? Instead, I get to become the master of getting a wheelchair up a steep driveway—at least I get my workout in. Although having my life threatened by the mom-in-law isn't fun.*"

It was so wonderful to have so much support. It is my belief that attitude can drastically change the situation, but reality can still end up horrible. We knew it did not help to sulk or feel sorry for ourselves, because it would just worsen the situation.

I was told we were in an exclusive club. Usually exclusive is used in a positive light but not in this context. This is not a club I would have preferred to be part of, but in hindsight I have met many wonderful people, and for that I am thankful.

The next day, Josh came back to the hospital and we had so much to learn and navigate. The nurses in the oncology unit understood the huge change that families experienced, and knew how to just be there for us. In general, nurses are unbelievable, but these nurses were extremely special. They knew that not just the patient needed a lot of care, but the families also needed understanding and support. They also knew that a new patient's family needs to learn a lot about things they don't know and wish they never knew. Fairfax Hospital has a whole team to help out a family that has to navigate through this new chaos. We met a child life specialist, which is a career I fortunately didn't know existed before this but am extremely thankful for. Our child life specialist's name was Holly. To meet Holly was truly a treat; she is this fun, amazing person, and once we found out she would be around to help us navigate through this unknown territory, it was calming. She focused on everyone — my parents, my in-laws, the rest of the family, and ourselves. I really do not know what to say about her, because I truly think words cannot be used to describe how an unrelated person can feel like family so quickly. When we had to go to the hospital, our first question was always, "Is Holly working? There was also a social worker assigned to us at the time, but she always seemed very uninterested and distant. I remember being at home cleaning Iliana's room to prepare for her arrival and to find a place for the multitude of gifts she received from our friends. Josh called me from the hospital to explain some things the social worker told him. I was angry with her because she seemed so uncaring. I honestly don't remember what she told Josh, but I recall being mad at her. I really only wanted to work with Holly. Holly had to tell us some uncomfortable things, but she did it in such a way that we knew it was going to be okay. I am glad we don't have to go to the hospital anymore, but I do miss her— everyone does.

5

First Days in the Hospital

Even though I still remember hearing Iliana's diagnosis like it happened yesterday, the raw emotions are better chronicled when they were actually felt. Most of the remainder of the book will be posts that were written by Josh and me in CaringBridge and on our Facebook page. The actual posts are italicized, with additional commentary in between.

Update 7/23/15

Iliana underwent her first spinal tap as well as the installation of a port in her chest to deliver her IV meds and to take blood. She came out of surgery like a champ and has had her first initial chemo treatments.

Words cannot express how we are feeling right now, but thanks to our wonderful family, friends and colleagues that have already formed what is now being called Team Iliana, the light at the end of the tunnel would be nearly impossible to reach. For that and the future support we receive from you, we are eternally grateful.

Thanks again for your support,

Josh, Gina, Sarah, Ithan and, of course, the captain and MVP of this team...Iliana

Update 7/24/15

Today, Iliana seemed to be her normal self, ignoring the people that are talking to her and not really caring about what they have to say, including the wonderful doctors and nurses that have been taking care of her. In fact, the oncologist that did most of the work on her so far said "this is going to be a wonderful two and a half year relationship." Her biggest issue is taking medication orally as she cannot stand the taste of them, but she has been a trooper in getting them down thus far. Thank God one of them is scheduled to be stopped on Sunday, assuming she continues down this good path.

Thanks again for all of the cards, balloons, stuffed animals, etc. If someone could provide a U-Haul when we leave, that would be great :).

That's it for now. Until tomorrow.

Update 7/25/15

Great day for Iliana. She was very active today. Played a lot in the kids' playroom, did some puzzles and art activities, and even had some buggy rides out in the courtyard for quite a while. Started to have a little bit of a headache towards the evening, mostly because of some elevated blood pressure due to the medication (completely normal by the way..no need to worry), but

Nurse Erica (an amazing night nurse whom we loved) quickly took care of that and now the headache is gone and the blood pressure is back to normal. Her appetite is certainly there. It was mostly a soup night, consisting of both tomato and chicken noodle, but she also had a side of mashed potatoes, Nutri-Grain bars and ended with a Popsicle for dessert.

Hopeful for another good day tomorrow—which is also Mommy's birthday.

I celebrated my birthday at Fairfax Hospital, not the ideal place to start the final year of my thirties. However, in true Rubin-style, we toasted my day with great food brought by my in-laws and dessert by my parents. We went into the family room that we had associated with bad news. Luckily, now we were able to see it as a celebratory room. My kids decorated the room for my birthday and for one day we got to enjoy the hospital and just have fun.

Update 7/27/15

Iliana had another good day today. Woke up to good vitals and blood test results. Got up and walked around the floor in her new slippers and played and colored in the playroom. Had a couple of visitors, which was nice. Dropped one of the meds that was needed three times a day. Iliana is not big on taking meds by mouth.

Update 7/28/15

Today was a great day for Iliana. She has had a lot of visitors thus far, but today's visitor takes the cake. Harper the dog came to visit Iliana today. The dog hopped up on her bed and was such an uplifting spirit for Iliana. It made her day (also made Mom's day as well). Iliana continues to be in good spirits, and she is progressing well as each day goes by. As of today, Iliana is scheduled to be released from the hospital on Thursday.

Tomorrow is another day. Until then.

Update 7/29/15

Hopefully, today was Iliana's last full day in the hospital. Tomorrow she is scheduled to check out after a spinal tap and round of chemo. She was able to see her two favorite nurses. Ms. Lindsay and Ms. Erica have been tremendous. As much as we wouldn't want to wish this illness on our worst enemies, these nurses have made these past two horrifying weeks as comforting as possible. I am not sure that Iliana could have been treated any better and have received any better care than she has from the nursing staff, but these two in particular. Thank you, Lindsay and Erica.

Looking forward to checking out tomorrow afternoon. Until tomorrow.

Update 7/30/15

Today is discharge day—but not before a visit from some Disney princesses.

All vitals look good, spinal tap went well and today's chemo treatment seems to have gone well. Iliana is super excited to be going home and test out her new bed, and more importantly, go to the bathroom without an IV pole. She had been an unbelievable trooper through this all. What an unbelievable little girl she is. We are so proud of her.

A lot had to happen prior to discharge day: the house had to be disinfected, we had to understand what medicines to give her and when, what she couldn't eat, what medicines she couldn't take, etc. We were suddenly nurses, caretakers, teachers, and social workers, all while being parents. As a nurse, we had to know that she couldn't take Advil since it's a blood thinner. As a caretaker, we had to know that she couldn't do certain things for fear of disturbing her port. As a teacher, we had to ensure our family and friends knew the risks and proper protocol, in addition to acting as educators during her time off from school. As a social worker, we had to be there for our other kids and explain the situation to them. These times were difficult for us, and I was always stressed and worried. Josh always wanted to know, and still does, "*When do you stop worrying?*"

One of the biggest things for her was what she couldn't eat. She couldn't eat items with skins on like strawberries and unpeeled apples. She couldn't eat raw food, such as sushi, biltong, or raw eggs. Sushi was a favorite and biltong is South African style beef jerky that Zeida makes from scratch. Raw eggs are found in a surprising amount of food, such as Bubbie's caesar dressing and Oma's chocolate mousse. Bubbie makes the best caesar dressing and Oma makes amazing chocolate mousse. Mayonnaise also has raw eggs, but we didn't know at the time, and luckily it didn't harm her. Deli couldn't be bought at the deli counter because even though the individuals behind the deli counter are sanitary, they can't be watched at all times. We were extremely lucky since, at the time, Iliana's best friend's mom was in charge of our local Giant. She was able to ask a trusted employee, Kenny, to slice deli for us. As soon as he cleaned and sanitized the deli machine, he would slice our order and put it aside in the fridge. We were able to eat our deli without fear. Kenny doesn't know this, but he will always have a special place in our heart—not just for the 'safe' deli, but even more for helping us keep one more thing constant.

6

Accessing the Port — Sara Willis

No one should ever have to stay in the hospital for such a long time. And although we knew it wouldn't be the last hospital stay, our drive to Purcellville was filled with excitement because we were heading home.

The drive in our neighborhood was awesome, as we drove by some unbelievable handmade signs welcoming us home. I will say this many times, that even though this was a horrible time in our life, we are lucky enough to have such caring people in our lives. To add to it, Sarah and Ithan, with help from our neighbor, Hannah Delmonte, also made a huge sign that they hung over the garage welcoming us back. It was colorful, beautiful and such a wonderful surprise. Even though the sign itself was spectacular, the smiles on my kids' faces were even more heartwarming. Since this whole ordeal began, we have smiled but never a full-faced, genuine smile that encompassed our whole faces and filled our hearts with warmth. But today we smiled from the heart, as our whole family was together again at home, including our two dogs.

Our friends and family had started a Meal Train, and as a result, people from all over had signed up to provide homemade meals for our family. Admittedly, not having to worry about food was nice. It took a fair bit of stress off knowing that food was covered. We are lucky to have such a wonderful community and family that helped provide for us through the tough times.

Update 8/4/15

Today was tiring. Had her best friend over for a while and Iliana was wiped. After a little nap, it was time to celebrate Sarah's eleventh birthday. Happy birthday, Sarah. Nothing like a little cake and family to keep Iliana busy.

Iliana continues to do well and is taking her meds like a champ. Thursday is her first outpatient chemo treatment at the clinic. We'll keep you posted on her progress each week.

Thank you for keeping her in your thoughts and prayers.

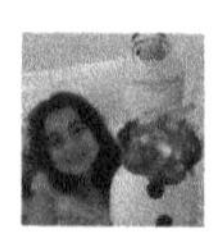

Iliana and a stuffed Olaf.

Update 8/6/15

Iliana had her first outpatient treatment today. Went really well. She was such a trooper getting the line put into her port. She will get used to it over time. While her general numbers look good, her ANC (the real white blood count that fights infections) is dropping as expected from the chemo. Unfortunately, this means that visitations somewhat come to a halt until her numbers come back up.

She continues to have a good attitude and has some brief moments of activity throughout the day, but it quickly catches up with her as you can see from today's picture. Good thing we have some really comfy chaise lounges.

Because of the steroids, she is eating anything that is not nailed down. Her favorite was Bubbie's lentil soup but now seems to be chicken nuggets, egg salad, bagels and Cheez-Its. She is drinking milk as if cows were becoming extinct.

All in all, she is doing great. I am of the opinion that she understands what is going on and is basically being herself in having an "I don't give a you know what attitude," which is perfect for her. Wouldn't want it any other way.

These updates may become more weekly as we go for her treatments. We will update with any important information. Big day comes in about two weeks when she has another bone marrow biopsy and spinal tap. This will show us how she is progressing and if she can move to phase two of the treatment cycle.

Thanks again for all the incredible support from all of you. It has meant more than words could ever express.

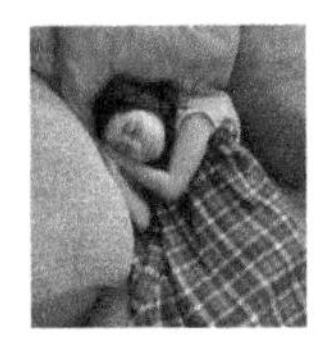

Accessing the port hurts. Even though there is a "hole" that is used every time chemo is done, skin is still pinched and broken when the port is accessed. It hurts but fortunately, one gets used to it as time goes on and it begins to feel like being pushed. The nurses and doctors assured us that at the end, Iliana will be a pro at getting her port accessed. Once again, this was reassuring that she would be okay with it. Looking around at the other kids, a connection was felt to the families. The clinic did their best to make this horrible experience as exciting for their little patients as they could. They have XBoxes, a teen room, as well as an art studio. This studio includes paints, markers, books, toys, etc., and our favorite, an art therapist — Miss Jess. Whenever we went to the clinic, Iliana always wanted to know if Miss Jess was there.

In the art studio, a child can paint a ceiling tile to hopefully inspire other children. When one looks up, they see amazing ceiling tiles, so colorful, beautiful and inspiring. Our favorite was painted by Sara Willis who had brain cancer and unfortunately lost her battle on November 22, 2018. This girl was inspirational. She fought cancer twice and became blind in one eye because of it. Instead of displaying defeat when she learned about her eye, she asked to be known as One-eyed Willy. James and Angie Willis raised such a beautiful and inspirational girl. Even with all these limitations and harsh obstacles, Sara kept smiling. Her obituary was very well-written and even though nothing on paper can define her amazing life, I am going to include it.

"*Sara was born on May 11, 2000 in Fredericksburg, Virginia. During her brief, wondrous life, Sara faced many challenges and she was renowned for tackling each with an infectious smile and a seemingly infinite amount of positivity. She lived passionately and joyously and loved to brighten others' lives through gifts, compliments and acts of kindness. Sara loved music and to dance and was often overheard saying, "dance like no one is watching." Sara's passing has left a massive hole in this world and our hearts. She will be greatly missed by all who knew and loved her."* She was eighteen at the time of her death.

7

Two Kids —Their Desire to Help

Second Visit to the Clinic 8/13/15

The past few days have been tough for our little fighter. The chemo is causing pain in her legs and walking is hard but she is pushing through. She was refusing to take any medicine that she didn't have to including Tylenol. We finally convinced her to take Tylenol, which will hopefully help alleviate her pain.

We had to go to the clinic today to get her last round of chemo for the induction phase of her treatment. Her counts were good, which is great news. Unfortunately, we also received some bad news. One of the tests they perform in the hospital is looking for any abnormalities with certain chromosomes. One of the tests found an abnormality (translocation of the twelfth and twenty-first chromosome). In layman's terms (or terms that I think I understand), she has to get treated as "very high risk" as opposed to "standard." This distinction means that regardless of the bone marrow results, she will have to go through more aggressive treatment in the next five months. The most important news is that the prognosis is still favorable and finding this now means she will be put on the right treatment path versus one that might not have completely eliminated the leukemia. In other words, today totally sucked! Let's be real, all of this sucks! But at least her prognosis is still favorable, her cancer is treatable and so we will continue to be positive one day at a time. We will shed more tears but we will laugh a lot! How can we not? With Ithan and his silly antics and Sarah and her contagious laugh, we are so fortunate to have children that see beauty and fun in everything. And of course, the leader of the pack. The one who refuses to give any doctor the satisfaction of a smile or even acknowledging his/her existence no matter how hard he/she tries. Her obnoxious attitude and her dirty looks help us know that she is going to be awesome! As one of Josh's friends said, " Cancer certainly picked the wrong girl to mess with!!"

My medical knowledge (which is extremely limited) on the various stages of leukemia and treatments are as such:

1 - **Standard - "low-risk"** = least aggressive treatment - cancer has a low risk of coming back.

2 - **"Aggressive"** = aggressive treatment - cancer has medium risk of coming back but side effects of treatment are more possible.

3 - **"Very aggressive"** = most aggressive treatment - if not treated vigorously, cancer has more chance of coming back.

I think I processed all of this but I still couldn't believe this was happening to us.

Another new thing I learned was that Iliana benefited from a clinical trial. So basically, a child who is "standard," such as Iliana, should have had a small chance of the leukemia coming back. However, it was found that forty percent of these kids were getting leukemia again. Scientists were dumbfounded at this high rate. They found that the kids who got leukemia again had a chromosome switch, specifically a translocation of the twelfth and twenty-first chromosomes. This means that in the first month, it is figured out which path to take, standard, high-risk or very high-risk, based on the genetics of the patient. As mentioned before, due to the translocation of these chromosomes, Iliana would have the very aggressive treatment to lower the risk that leukemia would strike again. Even though this path was harsh, it was preferable than even imaging that we didn't do everything as advised to try to keep this awful disease from returning.

While we were trying to process everything, so did our other young two. We were scared; they must have been terrified! They tried so hard to be good because the last thing they wanted to do was add more worry and pain in the family. I know of kids who act out because they are not getting as much attention as they used to, etc. Sarah and Ithan's response to sympathizing about Iliana's diagnose was the following:

Sarah and Ithan's Lemonade Stand and Bakery

There are days when my faith in people waivers and I wonder what is wrong with society. Fortunately, those days are few and the events of the past few days have definitely restored my faith in humanity. On Wednesday, Sarah and Ithan decided that they wanted to sell lemonade to benefit leukemia awareness. Thanks to some very generous neighbors, they made one hundred dollars. But that was not enough for my two philanthropists. They wanted to raise more money. So yesterday, they expanded from a lemonade stand to a lemonade stand and bakery (thanks to cookies made by Grandma). Our awesome neighbor contacted the local fire department, which put the word out about Sarah and Ithan's lemonade stand. Word started getting around about what these two were doing in honor of their little sister. The wonderful and generous individuals at Carlyle and Anderson came by with a very generous donation. Our heroes, the tremendous individuals who risk their lives for us (the volunteer and paid firefighters of Hamilton and Purcellville), came for a refreshing glass of lemonade. We even got a special treat when the firefighters raised the ladder for us. And of course, the unbelievable community of Purcellville and our outstanding neighborhood of Wright Farm who have already opened their arms to us and for us. You came by as well to help raise money for such a great cause (we can't forget all the help we got from our little neighbor friend (lugging the lemonade is hard work!!)). Our family - your support has made this unbearable experience bearable. As if you haven't done enough, you came by again. Because of all of you, Sarah and Ithan will be able to donate over eight hundred dollars in support of leukemia awareness and research. And they aren't done! Sarah's goal is one thousand dollars. Even Iliana is in on the action. She got one dollar from Zeidie today and turned around and gave it to Sarah and Ithan "for leukemia."

If I haven't said it, thank you. Thank you for putting a smile on Sarah and Ithan's faces. Thank you for making them feel so special. They have taken this tough time in our family and turned it around into something so great. And everyone's kindness and generosity has certainly inspired them. My two busy bees who worked from ten to four on Wednesday without a break can't wait to do it again. So tell your neighbors and your friends,cuz Sarah and Ithan's lemonade stand will be open tomorrow (Friday) from eleven to one.

With love.

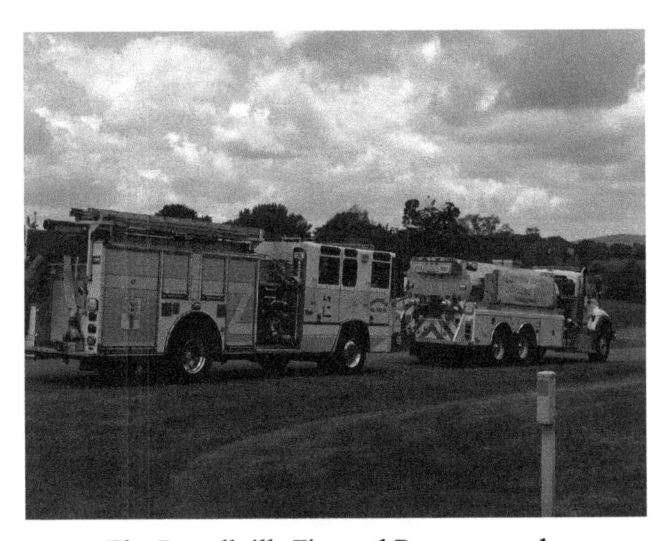

The Purcellville Fire and Rescue squads.

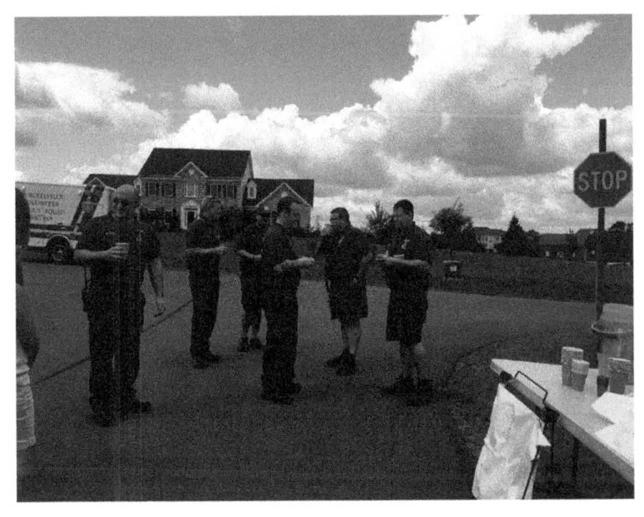

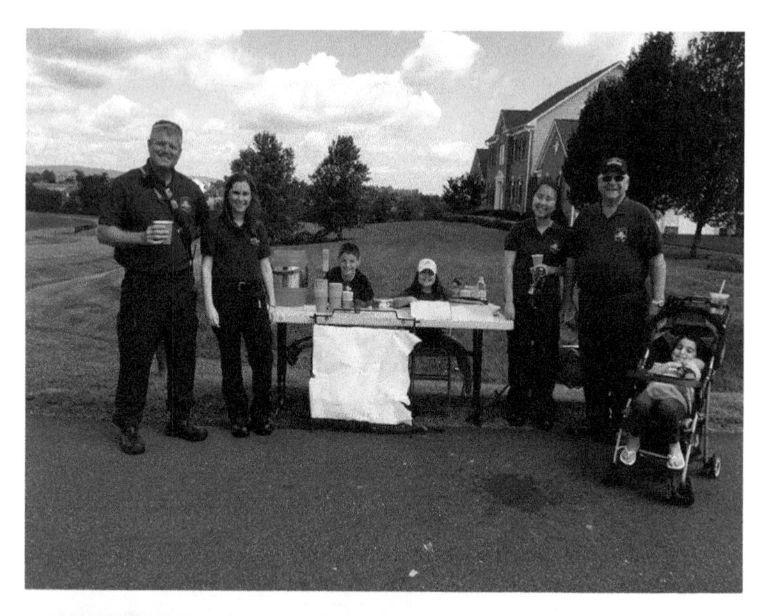

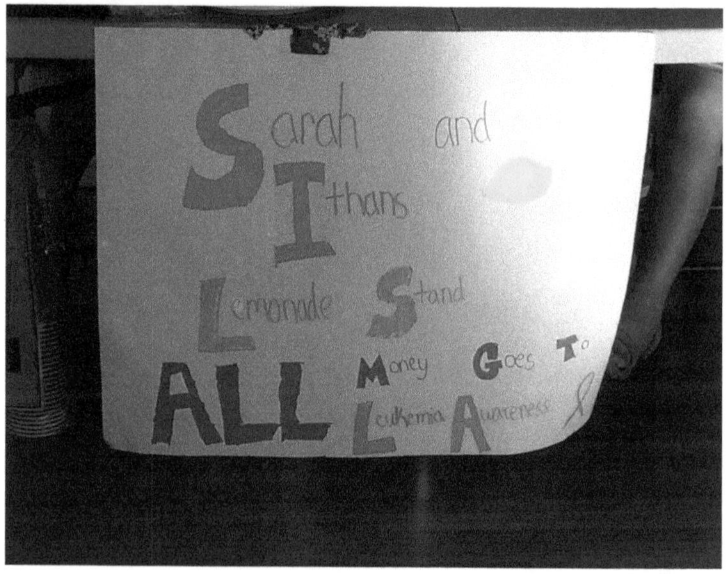
Sarah and
Ithans
Lemonade Stand
ALL Money Goes To
Leukemia Awareness

Two kids, a lemonade stand and their goal

It takes a village, a community. We all know that and once again we experienced how great our community, our little Mayberry, town of Purcellville is. Sarah and Ithan had raised eight hundred dollars between Tuesday and Wednesday. They wanted to raise at least one thousand dollars. Josh and I warned them that they probably wouldn't experience the same kind of activity and boy were we wrong!! Once again our town came through. Not only did they raise two hundred dollars on Friday morning but our very own Dragon Yong In invited them to set up their lemonade stand in the evening. The kids raised another four hundred dollars. So not only did they meet their goal but they exceeded it!!! Thanks to all the generous people who surround us and the amazing community who looks out for us, the kids will be donating over fifteen hundred dollars for leukemia awareness in honor of our beautiful Iliana.

A family friend of ours told me that Sarah and Ithan inspired her three kids to create a lemonade stand of their own. They had a stand at a bike path near them and also raised money for leukemia awareness. This horrible achiness in my heart was overwhelmed by the amazing spirit everyone was displaying.

Besides what the kids did out of the goodness of their hearts, there are so many amazing organizations for cancer. A lot are born out of the unfortunate knowledge of the Hell that cancer patients go through; others are created because they see first-hand the terrible suffering that this disease causes. Listed below are some of the incredible charities that exist in the D.C. area:

Team Mathias - the mission of Team Mathias is to

help support families and research efforts while raising awareness for ALL childhood cancers (taken from the Team Mathias website). We received a big box of goodies for all the kids specific to their tastes. Unfortunately, Team Mathias was founded because Mathias who was only eleven, was diagnosed with osteosarcoma, cancer of the bone, in July 2012. He passed away at the age of thirteen.

Stillbrave - Stillbrave's mission is to provide non-medical, supportive care to children with cancer and their families (taken from the Stillbrave website). Stillbrave was formed because at sixteen, a beautiful young lady named Shayla found out she had stage four Hodgkin's disease and died on January 28, 2009. She is the product of her father, Tattoo Tom, who is named that because he has tattoos all over his body. When he finds out a child has cancer in D.C., if he can, he comes in with a backpack full of Beanie Babies. A child picks a Beanie Baby of choice and is very endeared by this stranger. Then he provides the child's family with their own backpack full of necessary items that will help a child with his/her cancer treatments.

Smashing Walnuts - Smashing Walnuts was started because young Gabrielle was diagnosed with DIPG (diffuse intrinsic pontine glioma) – an inoperable brain tumor, which is terminal upon diagnosis. This organization provides funding and lobbying and directs resources to develop better treatment protocols and a cure (taken from the Smashing Walnuts website).

Ellie's Hats - Jay was a teacher for the Fairfax County Public Schools who founded Ellie's Hats because he noticed one of his students, Ellie, loved wearing hats especially after she lost her hair after being diagnosed with leukemia. Their mission is to brighten the day of children with cancer by sending them colorful and gorgeous hats.

LLS (Leukemia & Lymphoma Society) - LLS was created by the Villiers family in 1949 in New York because their sixteen year-old son, Robbie, died from leukemia in 1944. Dedicated to curing leukemia, lymphoma, myeloma, and other blood cancers, LLS is the world's largest voluntary (nonprofit) health organization dedicated to funding blood cancer research and providing education and patient services (taken from the LLS website).

Make-A-Wish - Make-A-Wish isn't specifically for pediatric cancer, it is for all children diagnosed with critical illnesses. A wish come true can be a crucial turning point in their lives. A wish can be that spark that helps these children believe that anything is possible and gives them the strength to fight harder against their illnesses. This impact is why Make-A-Wish is driven to make every one of these wishes come true (taken from the Make-A-Wish website).

All these organizations and many more reached out to us to help try to make our suffering easier.

8

Pancreatitis

Back to the Hospital We Go

Iliana was experiencing really bad stomach pains. We were told to bring her to the ER. One side effect of the chemo is high blood sugar and in rare cases, pancreatitis. Iliana has both. So if my accountant brain understood, the medicine caused the pancreatitis, which caused the high blood sugar. She now has what we hope is "temporary" diabetes. We will be here for at least a week, first in PICU for a couple of days and then back to visit our friends in the oncology unit.

If I meet another type of "ologist," I will have to be moved to floor four, which is the psychiatric ward.

This might be our second home for now, but we will be home soon.

Our stays at the hospital were always scary, but so far, this had been extremely terrifying. We didn't know what the future held for us, and first we had to inform our six-year-old that not only does she have leukemia but now she also might have diabetes. Our life was in such turmoil already, we couldn't have imagined it getting worse, but it did. We were doing what we could to cure her, but she received a medicine that we were unaware she was allergic to — Pegaspargase. This just felt like one step forward, two steps back. I honestly couldn't even fathom how our nightmare could get worse, but it just became a night terror.

Even though my heart was hurting from this, my head kept reminding me that Iliana was tough and stubborn. I never felt pessimistic about her life until this week. Throughout the few weeks after learning about her diagnosis, there was always light in her eyes, hope. She would always struggle when they had to take her blood through an IV. In the middle of her stay in the PICU, she didn't fight when they took her blood. She was so lethargic. I looked in her eyes, and they were tired. I think that was the first time I felt totally defeated. This whole scenario was an awful nightmare, but that day I just needed to sit, be away from all the misery, and cry alone. But I still had to be strong, show Iliana that no matter what obstacle was thrown at us, we would find a way to survive.

Hospital update 8/16/2015

Iliana is doing well. Her sugar level is normal, and her sodium is back to the right level. Our biggest concern throughout the night was that her blood pressure remained low. The doctors thought it had to do with her body being so dehydrated. We met a new "ologist" last night, a cardiologist. We got rid of him pretty quickly as fortunately, her heart looks great. It took a while, but early afternoon, her blood pressure stabilized and her heart rate went down. So now the next thing is waiting for the pancreas to settle down so she can eat on her own. We will have to continue with the insulin and the sugar checks for an undetermined amount of time until we know if her body can make the insulin on its own. She looks a lot better, and I saw a glow of Iliana when I suggested we brush her teeth and she gave me a dirty look. It was beautiful :)

Yesterday's Frustrations, Today's Happiness 8/18/2015

Yesterday, once again, proved to be a tough day. We were so happy as her numbers kept improving and she was starting to feel a little better. Until we noticed that her breathing patterns changed. A chest X-ray and ultrasound showed that she had fluid right outside her lungs. The ultrasound showed that it was a moderate amount of fluid. As of now, we are going to see if her body takes care of it. We will know more as time progresses.

Today, she has improved quite a bit. She was out of her bed, hanging in a chair. She was able to get off the insulin drip for a while because her sugar level dropped. Unfortunately, they had to start it again as they don't want to mess with her levels. Her pancreas is still healing and she hasn't eaten yet so once her pancreas is totally settled, we hope to get rid of the insulin.

That's the medical update; time for the attitude update:

It's back!! She is allowed one ice chip every ten minutes. And it is ten minutes on the dot!! The General, your Highness, or the Ice Czar are all applicable, as you better jump up and give her her ice chip on the dot. In fact, it's almost time, so I better get ready to hop to it!

Popsicle Heaven
8/19/2015

Never has a popsicle tasted so good!!!

We got the go-ahead to start clear fluids and see how she takes it. Once Iliana heard the word popsicle, she perked up and gave us a beautiful smile. She had enough of a popsicle to show off her red tongue but then decided that the popsicles here were not up to par. So we switched to apple juice. Word is that apple juice makes her tummy feel better. So far, she is reacting well to the fluids but we are taking it very slowly.

The fluid around her lungs seems to be going down. Her breathing is much better. But we still have a little ways to go. We pray that we continue to move in the right direction.

Iliana had a visit from a couple of princesses who gave her seashells and a necklace. :)

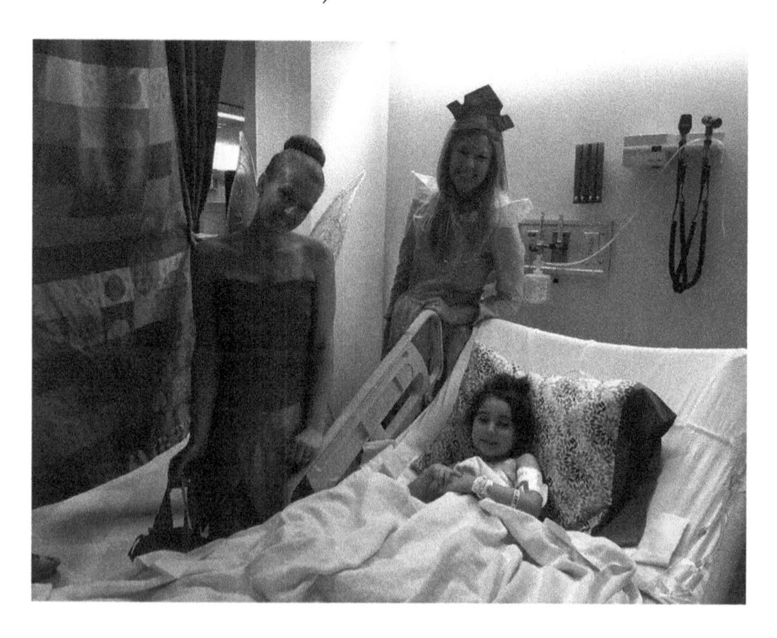

Her doctor thought that would be a good time to sneak up and try to catch a smile from her but he was mistaken. He got a dirty look. :) Such a busy morning, so I thought it was time for a nap. Apparently, I was mistaken; it is popsicle time. Hope to keep posting more good news.

Now that she was able to tolerate clear liquids, we went from the PICU to the oncology unit. When I close my eyes, I can still remember that room vividly. I think that's because even though every visit was tough and every room reminded us about Iliana's condition, that room was filled with some hope. The PICU in Fairfax Hospital at the time was not a place that was warm and welcoming. The toilet was in a cabinet, and it had to be pulled out to use it. If we needed to shower, we had to go to a family room down the hall. We kept Iliana's showers to a minimum, and something like going to the bathroom for her was a humiliating experience.

Besides the physical aspects of being in the PICU, the emotional part was even worse. Poor babies crying from pain, nurses scurrying around trying to do everything, machines beeping, and hollering through the night. This was the first time through this whole body-numbing experience Iliana looked tired. Her eyes lost all hope and for the first time, I was scared my little one lost all faith and wouldn't fight. She was so lethargic that she didn't even battle to have her blood drawn. It was the most awful, out-of-body experience ever. I think it was even worse than learning about her horrific diagnosis.

It was probably a contributing factor to my meltdown. I thought I was fine, but I was yelling at everyone, even the poor doctors and nurses who were just trying to help. I would like to say, it is understandable given the circumstances, but no one deserves to be treated or spoken to the way I vocalized myself. I am sorry to those who got the brunt of my frustration.

So Close, Yet So Far Away
8/25/2015

Sorry it has been a while since we updated everyone. This past week has been very difficult, filled with ups and downs and tremendous emotion. Thursday, Iliana got her last round of chemo for the induction phase and they checked her bone marrow. The doctors also released fluid that had collected around her left lung. Unfortunately, this caused air in her lung, so they had to go back in and put a chest tube in her to help release the air and any more fluid. Her electrolytes, magnesium levels, sodium levels and glucose levels still needed to be corrected. We still didn't know if all this caused permanent type 1 diabetes or if it was temporary. There was so much going on, but she took it like a champ. Her stomach still hurt but fortunately, pain medicine was able to alleviate her pain.

After her treatment and chest tube procedure, Iliana was pretty sleepy and just done with all of this. We saw glimpses of her old self at different points in the week but in general, her mood has been pretty down. The highlight of the week was when some of the wonderful teachers and our principal from our school came to visit her. They brought her a little crocodile, which is the symbol of our school. She smiled and spoke to them. It was wonderful. Even Ithan and Sarah were soooooooooo excited. (See, Mrs. Brownell, he is all ready to go back to school. :))

Emotionally, this week has been really tough for me. I am

told that I need to talk and reach out but it isn't that simple. I have to be strong for my kids and I am fortunate to be around them all the time. I don't want them to see me cry because I don't want them to think that everything won't be okay. Thursday was the day I needed time to myself. Where I needed to scream, yell at the doctors for not fixing her faster, and just cry. Asking why did it have to be her, wondering what was the reason that my little girl has to go through this. Why do my other two have to watch their little sister fight the battle of her life? How come I am missing some of my heart because I feel a piece breaking every time she cries or yells out in pain. Or even worse, when it looks like my little fighter has lost the fight in her eyes because she is so tired. Saying what a lot of parents say as they fight with their children — why us! it isn't fair. Of course, you don't want anyone to go through this. I pray for the day when I groan because it is 5:30 and I have to jump up and get ready for work. When I have to scurry around to get the kids off to school and rush home from work to get the kids to practice, etc. When I have to figure out how we are going to get laundry done and go grocery shopping because we have football on Saturday and baseball on Sunday. But I know that day will come. We will get there and with all the help from our family and friends, this will be a more manageable trip.

We did find out the best news possible on Monday morning. Her MRD came back negative, which means that the bone marrow test detected less than one percent of leukemia. In other words, the leukemia is gone from her body!! I almost tackled the doctor when she told me. It was much needed good news and the best news. We still have to go the Very High Risk path because of her chromosome abnormality, but this was still a huge deal!! Finally, I felt like we won a battle, won the game, and even though there were still plenty of other things to beat, we were getting closer to the Stanley Cup. And with all of our fans and my assistant coaches (Ithan and Sarah) and co-head coach, there was no way we weren't going to skate our way to victory (which is unlike any Washington team). And of course, our MVP was going to lead the way. The fight will come back in her eyes and nothing will stand in her way. So watch out leukemia, watch out cancer, and watch out Dr. Shurrin. :) Cuz as mentioned before, "cancer picked the wrong little girl to mess with"!!

At our Igloo :)
9/3/2015

We finally came home on Friday! I am not sure who was happier — me or Baxter/Annie. Iliana said she was, but her lack of emotion showed otherwise. I think her little body has been through so much that she is just tired. She still is not able to walk on her own and cries every time we get her to walk. Her feet are two and a half sizes bigger than usual due to swelling. We are so fortunate that our friends and great neighbors, the Bundicks, gave us some shoes that came in very handy. Her stomach has gone down, which is wonderful, and her pain in her belly is starting to subside. In fact, last night was the first night in a few weeks that Iliana has slept through. Both Josh and I were thrilled not only because we are actually able to walk straight but also because her belly and body are starting to get back to normal.

Next steps — Even though Iliana is still recouping from pancreatitis, we moved on to the next phase of chemo or the consolidation phase. This is a two-month period and I believe the toughest. She gets chemo everyday for the first two weeks in different forms and then I believe we go to the clinic twice a week for the last two weeks. The first month, she gets a spinal tab once a week and chemo via IV four times a week. She also takes chemo in the form of a tablet. Tuesday of this week was a long and tiring day, but fortunately it is only a once a week occurrence for the next two months. Tuesday, one of the IV chemos required tremendous hydration before and after the chemo. We left the house at 7 a.m. to make our 8:15 appointment in the clinic in Fairfax. We were there until 2:30 and then off to the hospital for her spinal tap, post fluid hydration and a blood transfusion. One of her protein counts that helps to absorb fluid was low. We finally got out of there at 8 p.m. and home by 9. I don't know how families do this that don't have parents, family, and friends who help however possible. We had Uncle Ezra come to put Sarah and Ithan on the bus, Mama Rosie picked them up from the bus, Coach Owens took them to practice, and then Bubbie picked them up from practice and fed them.

Iliana also had physical therapy on Wednesday to help get her walking and moving around again. Hopefully, this will help get her active again and feel better and somewhat normal. She has three more sessions scheduled, and we will see if we need any more.

We had a wonderful visit from one of my best friends from NYC, Mechal, and her husband, Chaim. They came with food, prizes and all around great spirits. Everyone should be lucky to have a Mechal and Chaim in their lives, as they only make it better. Apparently, my Sarah is trying to hijack Mechal as she talks to her every night. :) And the two of them designed the gorgeous shirts worn by my goofy models below. They are amazing!

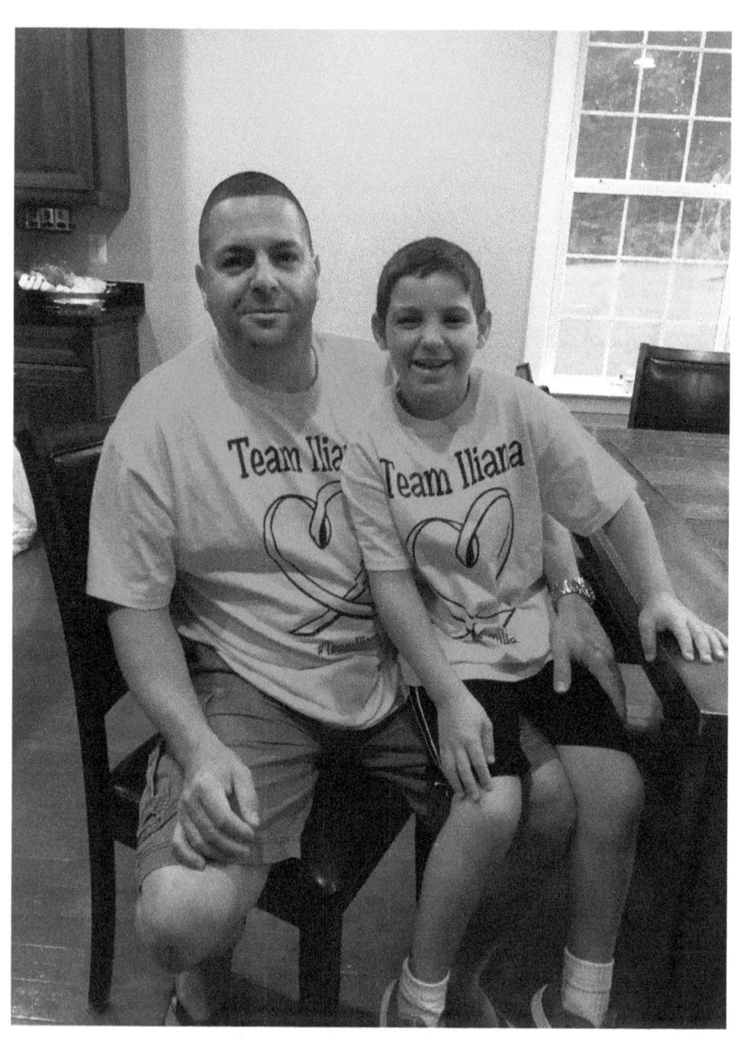

Uncle Ezra and Ithan sporting their Team Iliana shirts.

9

School Starts — Not for Everyone

School is Back in Session - a Bittersweet Experience

We started school on August 31 just like most of our friends. It was beautiful seeing all the back-to-school posts, but boy was it also sad. We could have posted pictures of two very gorgeous children going back to school with their big, beautiful grins and excitement and anxiety of what the school year would bring. Would Ithan love his teacher as much as last year? Sarah — how would middle school go? Would she be able to make new friends? How hard would the classes be? If anyone knows my Sarah, they know that all these fears were silly as she would attack middle school in the same amazing way she attacks everything else.

I didn't post. How could I post two, but not the three. Iliana will be joining her second grade class hopefully the beginning of next year. She has an incredible teacher and an incredible home-bound teacher. But it was hard to see all the other posts. I loved them, as I love seeing how great and beautiful everyone looked and how much they have grown. But it was bittersweet. I had two who were so beautiful and eager and one who looked so sad.

However, I am looking forward to next year, where I get to post my three. Ithan will have a big smile as now he will be ruling school — a big fifth grader. Sarah will be calm and cool, cuz now she is going into seventh and she will have the middle school thing down. And of course, Iliana — who even though she will still be in the middle of treatment will be wearing a big smile entering third grade.

But it is okay, maybe my first day post will come next year when Iliana heads back to school and I get to have three eager children heading to school, together.

Her second grade teacher was Mrs. Music. She was incredible. She allowed Iliana to talk to her class on her birthday so they could sing "Happy Birthday" to her. She also communicated well with Iliana's homebound teacher, Mrs. Goff. Mrs. Goff is special to us; she taught all three of the kids' first grade years, and even though she isn't a regular homebound teacher for Loudoun County schools, she had become one just for Iliana. She came to our house after school and taught Iliana what she needed to know so when she went back to school, she could easily be a part of the class. It was so special for Mrs. Goff to do that as it was one less thing Iliana would have to adjust to.

Birthday Girl

Today, our little warrior turns seven. She has been through so much in such a short time and has a ways to go, but a breakthrough smile today opened up some clouds. May your birthday be as bright as that beautiful smile. We love you!!!

Thanks again for all the incredible support from all of you. It has meant more than words could ever express.

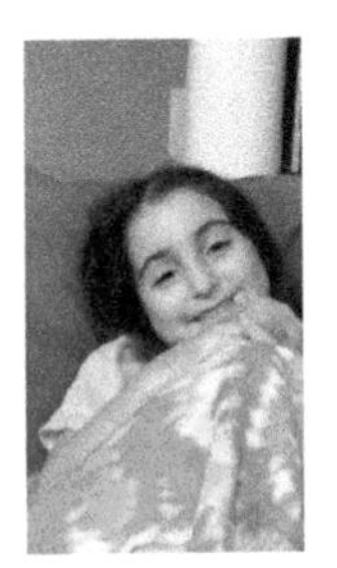

Part Two

My Daughter Saved My Life

10

When Lightning Strikes Twice

The month was September of 2015 when my world came crashing down again. I remember Ithan was playing football for our recreation league, known as the ULYFL, or the Upper Loudoun Youth Football League. We have always loved this league. Ithan was playing for the Bengals, the same team Iliana cheered for the year before, and Ithan had decided previously that this would be his last year playing football.

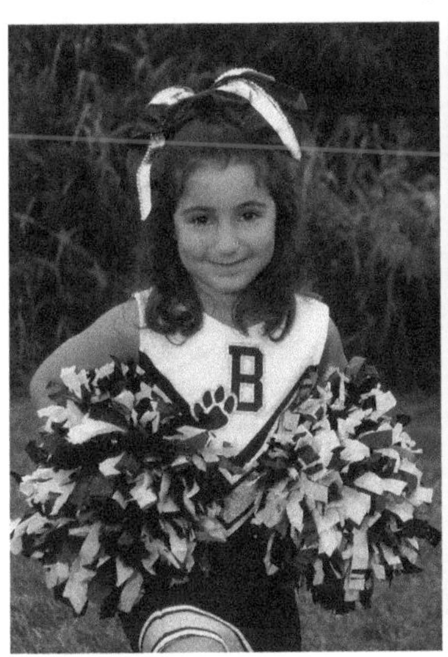

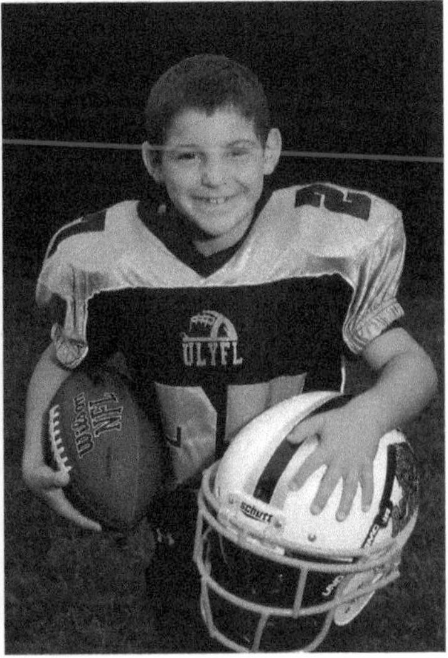

I wanted to be at all his games, especially because this would be his last year. Ithan wasn't the greatest football player, but he was still an athlete. He was the backup quarterback for the Bengals. The way the league used to play was that they allowed the less dominant players to play in the second quarter of the game. So that quarter, he played QB while the starting QB took a break.

I remember my parents or in-laws would stay home with Iliana, since Josh was a coach, so that I could go to Ithan's games. I remember taking Sarah to one game, played at our hometown field, Fireman's Field to be specific. The first quarter, I was in a lot of pain. I thought maybe I pulled something walking toward the field. I was in so much pain that I couldn't stand up to cheer on Ithan's team.

The second quarter, I still hurt, but my attention was on Ithan. So I ignored the pain and cheered him on. During halftime, I thought the pain would go away. After the third quarter started, I was so sore that I called Sarah over so that we could go home.

Luckily, the football field was only ten minutes away from our house. As soon as I got home, I collapsed into bed. My in-laws were kind enough to stay, so when Josh got home, my mother-in-law drove me to the Urgent Care five minutes away. I would have normally not gone but I was in so much pain that when I was told to get in the car, I complied. A quick exam didn't reveal anything, so the doctor prescribed me pain medicine and to follow up with my doctor. Mindy (my mother-in-law) dropped me off at home and went to fill the prescription. I was upstairs and the pain was so severe that I constantly asked if she was back yet. I wasn't trying to be a nag. I was just hurting so much that I just wanted the pain to subside.

Finally, Mindy got back with the pain medicine. I took it so fast that it could have been my first drink of water after days in the desert. Finally, the pain started to calm down and I went to sleep. This happened on Saturday. On Monday, I went to my doctor, who thought I might have kidney stones. Her thought was I should go to the urologist and the urologist should be able to prescribe something and give me helpful suggestions as to what to do to help manage the pain without having to take pain medicine. It would have been such a burden, especially now. In hindsight, kidney stones would have been annoying but better than my actual diagnosis.

I made an appointment at the urologist for the following Wednesday. The next Monday and Tuesday fell on Rosh Hashanah, an extremely important Jewish holiday, so no one was available until Wednesday. Until then, poor Josh would have to be the sole caregiver for the four of us. It ended up being good that my appointment wasn't until Wednesday, because Iliana ended up at the hospital. While at the hospital, I decided to go to the ER instead of waiting until Wednesday to go to the urologist.

If we hadn't been at the hospital, there is a possibility I would have not gone to the appointment on Wednesday. Maybe I would have been feeling better or Iliana needed me. My thought was that I would end up getting an X-ray at the urologist, but going would be such a nuisance because someone would have to be with Iliana, and we never knew when we would have to run to the hospital.

I knew it would probably cost more to go to the ER, but at the very least it would be done. We had both cars at the hospital, so the plan was that I would take the kids home and stay with them and then come back the next day to relieve Josh and he would go home. My in-laws were with us at the hospital, so Mindy came down with me to the ER. I anxiously waited my turn, as I just wanted a prescription and to go back up to Iliana.

Once I was taken and I explained my symptoms to the ER nurses and doctors, they ordered an X-ray for me. I was taken back to get X-rayed and even though no one could confirm, they felt it was cancer. I had two small tumors on my adrenal glands and one had burst, causing the pain. I thought I was dreaming. It wasn't possible. How could Iliana have cancer and now possibly me?

Random thoughts went through my mind, but the loudest one was how was I going to take care of Iliana if I was sick too. Receiving that kind of news is a blow to anyone, but knowing that my daughter was sick as well was mind-boggling. I was trying to fathom how my parents, husband, brother, kids and friends would have to hear this. Now it felt like Josh would have all the burden on him.

The fear of the unknown was scary. What treatment would I receive? Would I have to go to the hospital as much as Iliana? How would my body react? These questions, and many more, swirled in my head. The few days when I could not even get the energy up to help him prior to knowing why I was in such pain was torture for me not only physically but also emotionally. Here I was adding extra work to my husband's increasing workload — he had to take care of Iliana, the other kids, the house, dogs, work, everything else and now me. Luckily, I married a great, hard-working man who hardly ever complains.

As painful and awful as kidney stones are known to be, this was worse. Fortunately, going to the ER turned out to be the right thing. I was admitted, as they had to do a biopsy the next morning to confirm cancer and if it had spread. When I explained that Iliana was in the hospital also, they put me right above her on the ninth floor. I found out later that I should have been across the hospital in the adult oncology ward, but they knew it would be easier for myself, friends, and family if I was just an elevator ride away from Iliana. I really appreciate their sacrifice for me.

The next day, I got the biopsy under my arm, and the oncologist, Dr. Spira from Virginia Cancer Specialists, came to see me after the surgery. He told me that he would have the results in a few days. I begged him to call me with them. I could make the appointment, but because we might have to rush Iliana to Fairfax, I didn't know if I would be able to keep it. I know, this was my health, but the reality was that life still had to be dealt with — kids still had to be fed, picked up, and Iliana might have to go to the hospital at the drop of a hat. Once again, my focus was on Iliana, not myself.

Admittedly, I thought the reading of my X-ray was a mistake. It just wasn't possible that I could have cancer too. Doctor Gina apparently knew better than the nurses and doctors who had been practicing for years.

11

Confirmation

I was at work when I got the call confirming I had cancer. I could hear the pain in Dr. Spira's voice, because even though this life-changing message was one he delivered a lot, he rarely had to tell a mother whose daughter was also battling cancer. I remember just staring at my phone stunned. Even though I knew it was a probability that I had cancer, this was confirmation. Dr. Spira said I have lymphoma but there were a lot of types and he had to wait to get some more results before he knew what type I had. As of now, I could get my treatment at Loudoun,a closer hospital and clinic of theirs, but if it is more rare then I would have to travel to Fairfax for treatment. Their Loudoun office was still being established while the Fairfax one had been around for a while.

Having two of us with cancer was awful, but I am sure most people would have reacted like I did. I am not a saint, but worrying about others and not myself is who I am. I didn't think that my reaction was "special" but I am told it was. I still believe most other individuals in my shoes would have done the same. We did try to keep an upbeat house even though so much misery had befallen us and tried as much as we could to live a normal life even though our lives were far from it.

I also feel that after my initial reaction to such life-changing news dropped, I didn't react like a person hearing such scary news about her own health because of Iliana. I was not afraid of my own situation; I was more fearful of how it would affect my care of her and my other two. Of course, I was worried about my health, but even though my diagnosis was awful, I didn't allow myself to let it weigh me down or even think of it as significant as it was. My focus on her allowed me to not fear my diagnosis. I am sure my reaction would have been more intense and worrisome if she hadn't been going through her treatments at the same time.

Now, I had to tell Josh, my kids, family, friends and work. I needed to leave work, but I couldn't just leave and I couldn't tell them before I told Josh. So the only solution was to call Josh first. I asked my boss to come into a conference room so I could tell him about my diagnosis. After I told him, he sent me home for the rest of the day off. After I left work, I called my parents and was very matter-of-fact telling them. Again, I believe it is because of my concern and focus on Iliana. To me, this scary diagnosis was a real nuisance; now I would have to get chemotherapy, worry about getting sick and everything related to my care. I wouldn't be able to just drop everything and take Iliana to the hospital. Someone else would have to take care of her needs if I wasn't able to because of the chemo side effects or if I wasn't healthy enough.

Later, I asked Josh his feelings after I told him about me. He said:

"We were already at Fairfax Hospital with Iliana and you were still having side pains. During this time, you figured that you might as well get looked at while we were there to see if there was something other than a stone that Urgent Care at home told you it was. I honestly was thinking to myself as you went to the ER, "How am I going to handle two people in the hospital after you have surgery to remove the stone?" Jokingly, I said to myself, "Maybe Gina and Iliana can be roommates at the hospital." Never, for one second did I think that it would be something other than a stone; certainly, not cancer. Unfortunately, the latter proved to be the diagnosis. My wife had lymphoma. My first thought again was, why were they being punished? Why not me? How am I going to tell Sarah and Ithan? I have done things wrong in my life, but I try to be a good person who always tries to do the right things. Why do people like terrorists, killers, rapists, etc. get away with things, but my wife and daughter are sitting in a hospital bed being poisoned so that they can be cured of cancer? If I had any faith after my brother had died early in my life, it sure as hell was all lost after this. I don't believe that anyone in my family knows this, but I talked to Rabbis, Priests and others to get answers to Why? The best they came up with was the cliché statement that "God wouldn't give us anything that we couldn't handle." No one should have to handle anything like this. Not my wife, not my child, not my other children and not me. All faith was lost and now I just had to manage things the best way that I could. I had to make sure that my two "healthy" kids were taken care of and that their lives didn't change much, although that was damn near impossible. I had to find a way to work, take care of two cancer patients and my two kids. All I

can say is that I was a lucky man to have such great family, great friends and a fantastic community. They made the impossible, possible. I am forever grateful to them all for helping us out with whatever we needed. I am always reminded of how amazing I am for having pushed through all of these things without wavering and having continuous strength. That actually angers me. I don't consider myself amazing. I consider myself a husband and a father. I think any good father or husband would have done the exact same thing. There is no choice. Any less of a man does not deserve to be called a husband or a father. The true "amazing" husbands and fathers are those that have not only had to stay strong while their loved ones were undergoing cancer treatment, but those that have also had to stay strong for themselves and their families after their loved ones have died from cancer. I can't even begin to imagine how that is accomplished. It is funny, but I consider myself lucky. I know that sounds ridiculous, but if you put it into perspective, it is one hundred percent spot on."

My concern for Iliana and nonchalant reaction to my diagnosis can be seen in my blog. I devoted two paragraphs to her and casually informed people about my diagnosis. I had been diagnosed with Burkitt Non-Hodgkin lymphoma, a very aggressive form of lymphoma.

Iliana and I were driving down the road and she asked the most dreadful question: "Did I make you sick?" Such an innocent question but filled with a lot of anxiety and fear. What could I say to her to make her feel better and really understand none of this was her fault? I answered her the only way I could have thought of, with the truth. I wanted her to understand that cancer is not contagious and that cancer picks anyone it wants to no matter the person's race, financial standing, or values. None of this could have been avoided but all of it was painful and unfortunate. In fact, I think the opposite occurred. Had I not gone to the ER that day, and if I put off the urology appointment, I may have waited too long. In that way, Iliana having leukemia and being in the hospital the night I decided to go to the ER saved my life. So I say, "My daughter saved my life."

9/25/2015

Sorry it has been a while but it has been busy and tiring. A lot has happened since our last update:

1 - We have been to the hospital twice. The first time, Iliana wasn't feeling well and she weighed less than she weighed when she was initially diagnosed. So the doctors decided that she needed a feeding tube. This turned out to be a great decision as it has definitely given her strength and she is feeling better. She still isn't eating, which for this part of chemo is to be expected. We were in the hospital for about a week and unfortunately over Rosh Hashanah. We came home on the second day of Rosh Hashanah.

2 - We went back a few days later because Iliana had a fever. We ended up spending four days at our second home as Iliana had an infection. She is on antibiotics and looks to be feeling a lot better. The most significant part of our stay is that Iliana walked and stood up on her own!! She has not done that for a month and, of course, as you can imagine, we are so so thrilled!

But I am not done yet. Today Josh had to take Iliana back to Fairfax for a follow up and to get a new feeding tube. Her tube got clogged, and so he had to head back to the hospital to get it replaced. We pray that our next updates are all good news and encouraging words.

But don't worry, there is still more. I never had kidney stones. For some odd reason, I decided to go to the ER in Fairfax (hey, we were already there) and get myself checked as I was still having discomfort. If you know me well, I wanted them to take a CT scan and let me go upstairs so I could be with Iliana and they could call me with the results. They wouldn't. I found out that I have high grade Non-Hodgkin lymphoma. I will find out more next week, but I will get a port on Tuesday and Iliana and I will be twinsies. :) The treatment should only be for four months and I should feel better fast.

Thank you to all the families who have brought us dinner. It has helped us more than you can imagine. Thank you to our friends for their support and love and, of course, to our family; I don't know how we would do this if you weren't here. There are days right now where I believe our luck has run out. Wondering what did we do so wrong, that we need this kind of punishment. Then I realize that although this is horrible and life will be hard for the rest of this year, we really are still lucky. We live in a community that will drop everything to make sure we are okay and that our kids are happy. Adopted grandparents who come and clean for us and take care of us as though we are their own. I have a brother and sister-in-law that will be here in a second. And of course, our parents, who deliver chicken soup, drive us places, babysit, clean — do whatever is needed to make our lives easier.

Looking forward to a better fourth quarter.

I asked my close family and friends what were their thoughts when I was diagnosed. Mindy explained, "*I was driving and I called Josh to find out how everything was. He said, "Are you driving? Pull over and stop." Then he told me about Gina. I was speechless. I went numb. Then I realized I had to be strong for all of you and Dad.*"

Nona (Toni) said the following, "*It was a Thursday and I was in your kitchen mopping the floor when Mindy came in. I told her not to walk on the floor and she looked at me like I insulted her. She said, 'This is important." I then took another look at her and knew I needed to stop. We went into the family room. We sat together and she said, "It is not kidney stones; Gina has cancer." We cried together and held hands. I didn't know how to register this. I couldn't think how to make this better, how to help you. I said to Mindy, "She's in God's hands. The Blessed Mother will send her the strength, courage and endurance to get through this. And, she has you and Ron and her parents. Besides, she still has memories to make and she needs to dance at all her children's weddings."*

I went to Mass on Sunday and felt numb. I looked around and thought of the people there. What are they thinking? Who are they praying for? What are they enduring in their lives? I was angry with God that this has happened to this beautiful woman. Why was all I could think of saying. I thought, "You are such a coward that all you can think of is 'why?'" So I started to pray and pray hard."

Sarah told me she remembered that she, Ithan and Iliana were sitting on the couch in our family room when Josh told them about me. Sarah said she ran crying up the stairs to her room. My parents had just come to our house and my mom went upstairs to try to comfort her. She said, "*I recall sitting with Sarah, cuddling her, and Sarah being upset, and looking for reassurance...*"

12

Our Mayberry

Happy Days
10/13/2015

As most parents know, there is nothing more difficult than watching your child in pain. Seeing her lose her beautiful smile, missing her contagious laughter and temporarily losing her strength so she cannot stand or walk hits you in a place you didn't even know existed in your heart. But you as a parent have to find the strength to maintain your smile, faith, positive attitude. You have to know in your heart that you are doing the right thing to make your child better in the long run — no matter how tough the situation is now. And then there is nothing more wonderful and tremendous then when you hear her laughter again, when every day the beautiful smile is back on her face and she is trying to run around the house. The feeling you have when you see her playing with her siblings again, and see that mischievous smile, knowing that her brain is thinking up some naughty idea. I knew we would get here, I knew that we would have our amazing daughter back, but the few weeks when she was so unhappy, it was tough on us and the kids. But we toughed our way through it. Sarah took such good care of her, playing with her, trying to make her smile, and never gave up. Ithan with his goofy smile and silly antics kept me laughing, helping to keep me in good spirits. I can't say that life is easy yet or that we are done with the tough times. But it is better, laughter is back in the house, and we pray that we continue in this direction.

That being said, I have to admit, I do question my faith in God these days. It is hard to answer Sarah when she asks, "Why must Iliana go through this? She is so little; it is not fair!" In fact, last night I cooked a meal that mixed meat and cheese. (Josh was very happy. :)) (We don't mix meat and cheese per the Jewish guidelines we follow). I believe this is my way of rebelling. Of asking God what we did to deserve such a tough path. As I told the kids, I will always have faith and believe in God, because regardless of the tough months behind and ahead of us, I will always appreciate what we have: my unbelievable children, my amazing husband, our loyal and loving family, and our generous and amazing friends. And most importantly, the very positive prognosis for Iliana and me. I guess I had to do something to help me believe, to ensure that I don't lose faith. Perhaps, it is more important to be a good person as prescribed by most religions more than following the guidelines, because just following the laws doesn't mean you are contributing in a good way to the world. But that, of course, is a personal decision, one that every person has to evaluate on their own.

On a completely different note, I want to thank all the families who have brought us dinner. It has helped in more ways than you can imagine. And thank you to our sports' families who are always looking out for us and taking care of my boys. For proudly wearing Iliana's name on your chests and helmets. We love you so much for what you do for us.

Hoping to send out more good thoughts.

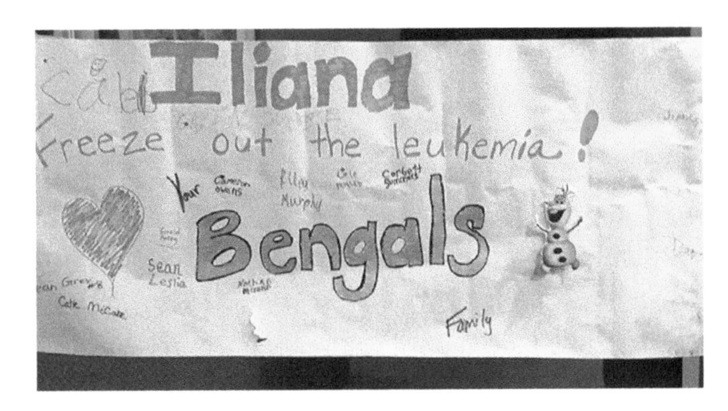

Our Bengal family representing the first game of the season.

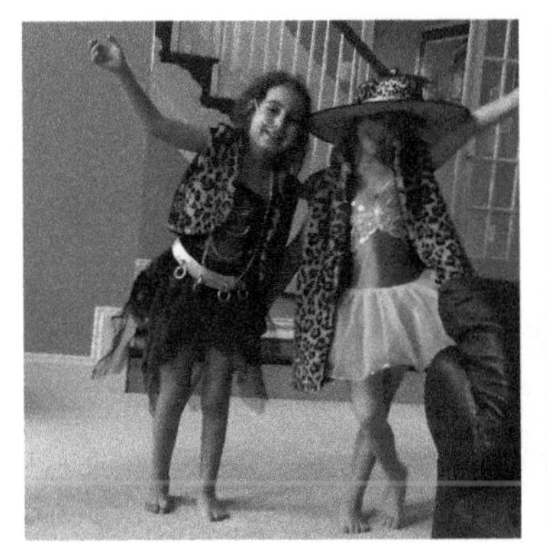

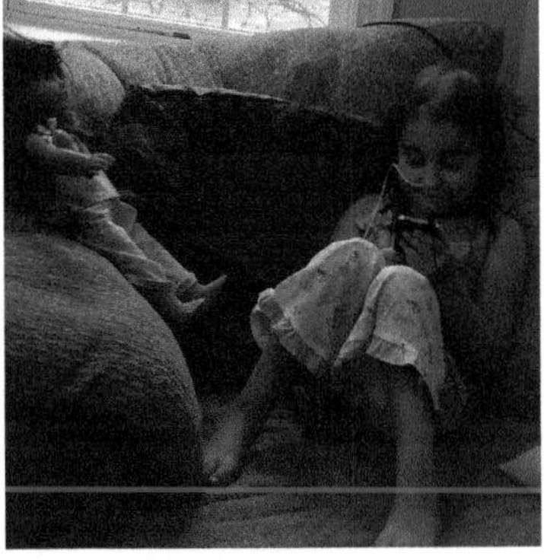

Left: Iliana and her best friend Ryleigh. Right: Iliana wearing her American Girl Doll PJs from Uncle Chaim and Aunty Mechal.

10/19/2015

There have been many nights in the past few months that I have cried myself to sleep. As you can imagine, a lot of tears were shed due to sadness, fear and terrified pure emotion. This past week, I went to sleep with teary eyes again. But this time, my tears were from joy, thankfulness, amazement! The beautiful words, kindness toward us and love that has been expressed and shared is overwhelming. The community that we hold so dear has embraced our pain as theirs and has taken the time to support us in any way possible. The dinners, the rides, the constant kind sentiments have meant more than I can ever express. I wish I could thank everyone personally but unfortunately, I can't. So please know that Josh and I are very grateful. We are grateful for the people who surround us, who we get to call friends. We are thankful for the strength that we get from knowing that we have the most unbelievable community supporting us. Even through this tough time, we feel blessed. We love our "Mayberry." And we will never forget what you have done for us and are doing for us.

Put your gloves on, Purcellville, cuz the Rubin girls will never stop fighting!

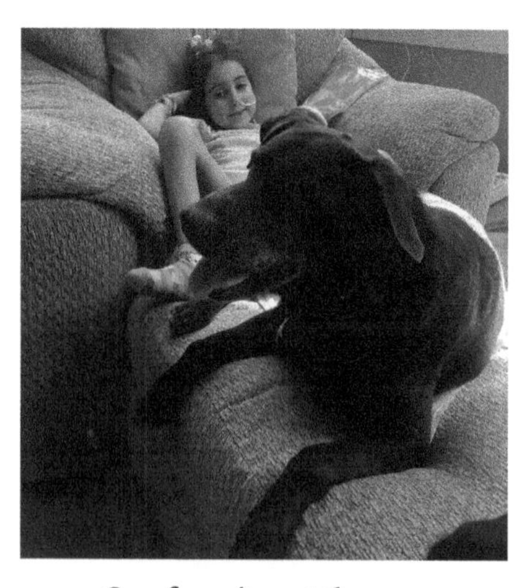

Our favorite pet therapy.

13

Don't Fear Striking Out — Play the Game

More Than Just the Game 10/22/2015

I have always loved spending my weekends on the football field or baseball field watching Ithan dive for a baseball or Sarah cheering for the Seahawks. Seeing such joy and raw emotion does not only become a wonderful memory but also a learning experience. Knowing how to lose or win gracefully is not always a natural reaction but sometimes has to be a learned attitude. This is some of what being a part of a team can teach everyone. Yet there is so much more than just the obvious; we have gained so many valuable friends throughout the years that have enhanced our lives more than I can imagine. What was a place for our kids to have fun and gain some valuable life lessons turned into our community. This past year, these generous families and leagues have taught us and our children an even greater lesson. Being part of a small town sports group is not just about the team and your friends, it is about the whole community, it is not just about the game but it is about what the game means and the knowledge that you are never alone.

This year, our Bengal team proudly wears a patch that has the initials IGR in pink with an orange leukemia ribbon. The boys are wearing orange socks and the girls are wearing beautiful pink and orange bows. As mentioned in an earlier post, our amazing team Mom made Iliana a beautiful banner that the whole team signed. Then some friends from another team duplicated the patches into stickers. These sentiments have brought so much warmth to our family. Every time I see the sticker or the patch, my eyes light up and my heart is warm. But the love and kindness doesn't stop there.

This past Saturday, our new dear friend, Coach Ro (Sarah's cheer coach from the Seahawks), taught the cheerleaders a special cheer to perform for Iliana at halftime. The end of the cheer, the girls made a heart with their pom poms and put Iliana in the middle with Sarah. The Seahawk football players and their coaches stood in a line behind the girls. After the cheer was done, the boys walked around the girls and gave Iliana a yellow rose with a blue ribbon tied around it. Head Coach Greg Caccavo — Sarah's science teacher as well:) — gave Sarah some roses. The game and halftime performance were dedicated to Iliana and everyone cheered her on. A few days have passed since this unbelievable display of affection, yet I still tear up and get goosebumps every time I think about it.

But wait, there's more!! As though this wasn't enough to fill my heart, our friends went even farther. They are doing a benefit for us at our beloved family sports bar, Coach's Corner, on December 5th. Our close friends are working so hard to put this on for us, our friends who we met through our different sports teams. They created a Facebook site, Team Iliana and Gina. Then the ULYFL, the football league that we play in, sent out an email supporting the event and showing us overwhelming dedication. I am so overwhelmed and floored by our friends, by our community. It is true that life has given us a tough path, but everyone who travels it should be so lucky to have the people that surround us. To be able to teach their kids the true meaning of being part of a team. That it is more than winning and losing, that it is really the camaraderie that is formed, the everlasting friendships, and just the joy of being part of something greater than yourself. I thank you, Upper Loudoun Sports, for showing my children what it means to be part of a community and for filling our hearts with warmth and love. And for making the football field more than just grass and cleats, but cherished, warm memories.

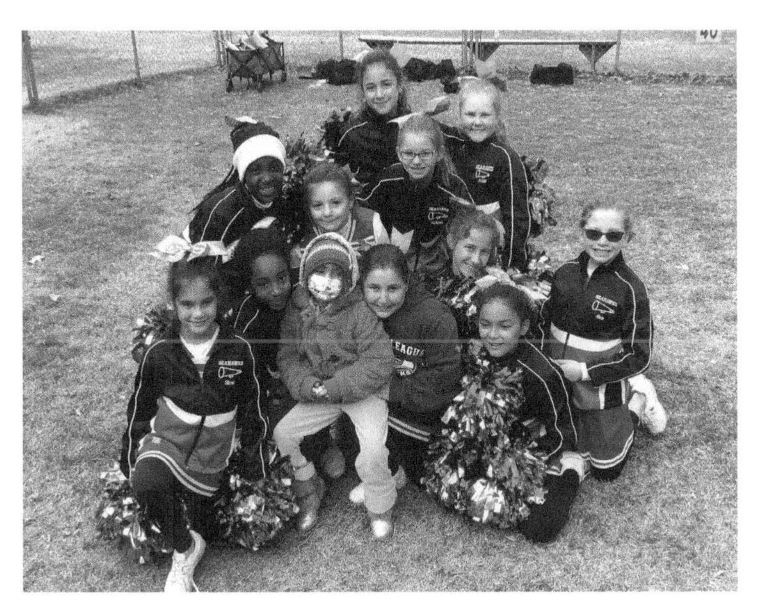

Iliana and the Seahawk cheerleaders.

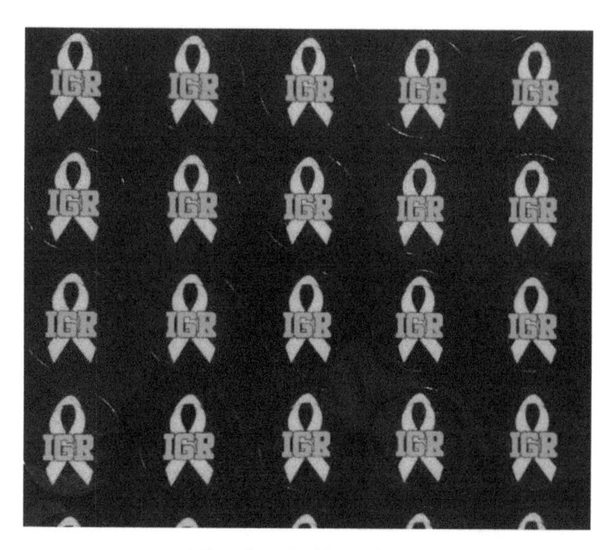

The football stickers.

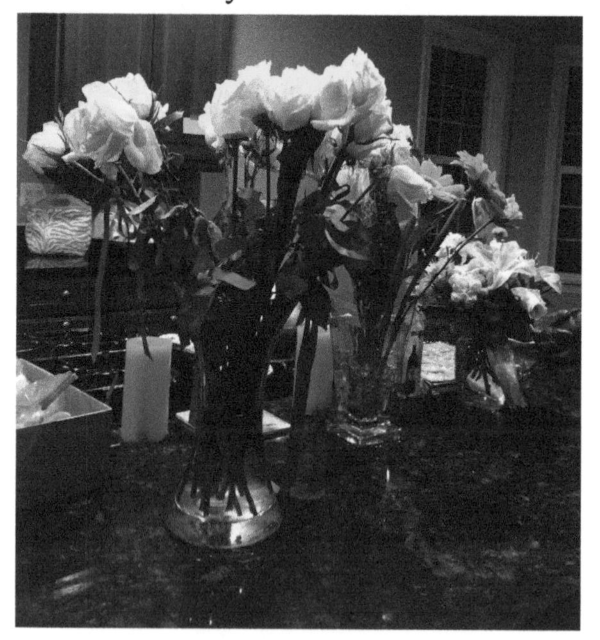

The Seahawk roses.

14

My Nephew's Moment to Shine

Bright Moments
11/20/2015

I am happy to say that it has been a while since I have updated our site. We have been busy almost being normal. Unfortunately, we are still running to the hospital and clinic, but fortunately it is for scheduled visits. Iliana's MRSA is gone and she has so much energy I can't seem to keep up with her. She is back to her old diva-self, the mischievous smile on her face, expecting her minions to do her bidding.

But today I write for a different reason. Last night, Iliana and I donned our new hairpieces to take pictures for a very exciting weekend, as this weekend my nephew will be a Bar Mitzvah. In the Jewish world, he is officially a young man. It was certainly a new experience for me, as I love my hair and not having it for what is such a momentous occasion in our family's life was certainly something I didn't expect. When we started discussing this wonderful tradition, I was probably annoyed that my hair was flat or not curly enough. Yet now, that doesn't seem to matter as much. Sure, I wish both Iliana and I could jump out of the shower and put a clip in, but that isn't our choice. We will throw on a hat or wear those silly wigs, which I have to admit I thought would be so easy to wear. I mean, really, I should have to just throw it on, but wow, it is so much harder than that. They have a mind of their own. The best part of all this though is the perspective that life forces you to see. Who cares about my hair or what I look like (well, let's be honest, I of course do) but more importantly is that both Iliana and I will be there to celebrate this wonderful occasion with our amazing family. I would have never anticipated that six months ago all I would want is for both her and me to feel good and have the energy to dance the night away. But this is where we find ourselves. And we both will. We will watch with pride as this handsome young man stands tall in front of his friends and family. We get to celebrate with him and enjoy every moment as a family should. I am so excited to be the proud Aunty (or Taine, as Ross calls me. He pronounces the yiddush word for Aunty as "tiny" as he is taller than me. :))

In addition, my brother and sister-in-law had so much to plan for the Bar Mitzvah. Yet they remembered every tiny detail in relation to Iliana and me. They worried where we should sit, is the food okay? They wanted to ensure that we would be able to be there, to partake in this exciting time even though they had so much to prepare and plan. I am so thankful for that. I knew I had a wonderful family; I am so proud to be a part of this family, one that I know will always be there for each other. I will watch with pride as this handsome man continues to make our family beam. I will laugh when he comes over to hug me, only because he is taller than me and he loves reminding me of that as he looks down. And I am sure I will cry when he hugs his little cousin who cherishes him and loves him as only the youngest cousin can love the oldest. And I will be thankful to be there, to enjoy the moments of this time. As a family, we will cherish this wonderful occasion and be thankful that we are all there together, breathing in what fun and exciting times life has to offer. As we have learned, life doesn't always allow you to dictate how you want to celebrate it, but you have to appreciate it for what it offers. And so we will.

Mazel tov, Ross! Thank you for bringing us this bright, shining moment. We love you!

We are very lucky as so much goodness was happening that holiday season. We had Ross's wonderful Bar Mitzvah to attend, the awesome fundraiser put on by our friends, and they were also doing a Sip & Shop to help raise money for us. The Sip & Shop was a bunch of different businesses that got together in one location, the house of our friends, the Kabbans. Mary Kay, Doterra and Lulu Lemon were only a few of the businesses represented. As if giving us the proceeds of their sales wasn't generous enough, some businesses also gave us items.

11/23/2015

As always, I tear up and say my blessings thinking of all that I have around me and the people we have surrounding us. This is well overdue, but I am so grateful for everyone who worked so hard to make the Sip & Shop a success. First, all the amazing women who came out to support us and make the event so wonderful and vibrant. To all of you, you are amazing!!! Thank you so much for your kindness, your generosity and your time. For those who I know, you understand how much you mean to me. To the lovely women I didn't have a chance to meet or thank personally, my heart is bursting. I hope that I get the opportunity to meet you one day in our beautiful town or maybe at the fundraiser. (I can't believe it is almost here!)

To Danielle Kabban, Brandi Payne and Tanya Owens, your friendship and your families already make our lives complete. (Your husbands definitely add so much color in our lives. :) Thank you for taking so much time out of your busy lives to do this for us. I hope that I never have the opportunity to repay you in this way, but I pray that even while we are old and gray, we will always be together.

With love

11/24/2015

My legs were hurting and my body was begging for rest :) Yet I would do it all over again. This weekend was incredible! My nephew became a Bar Mitzvah and did an unbelievable job. The best part was that Iliana and I were able to partake in all of the festivities. Friday night through Sunday! As I am sure you can imagine, this particular year was even more special. I didn't realize how moved I would be walking into the Friday night service. In usual late fashion —I had to fix that thing on my head :) — I walked in during the Rabbi's speech. He was talking about being thankful and the time of year and life. I sat there, tears in my eyes, because even though this is not how I imagined experiencing this wonderful event in my family's life, Iliana and I were experiencing it! We were living and would live! We were there and we plan on always being there. Man, I hoped that I would be able to manage through the rest of the weekend somehow not being an emotional mess!

We did. We listened as my nephew wowed us with his wonderful haftorah and everything else he did. I loved his connection with the Rabbi and Cantor and his religion. You could feel the family love and warmth and just the thankfulness.

And we danced the night away. But not before my brother and sister-in-law and nephew did a beautiful thing. First, my nephew wanted to paint his nails orange for his special occasion in honor of his little cousin. (Fortunately, his parents talked him off that ledge. :)). Then we were told that the money that would have been used for party favors was going to be given to Stillbrave. Stillbrave is an amazing organization that helps families who have children suffering from pediatric cancer.

My heart is full. Our journey is not an easy one right now, but it is still full of happiness and gratitude. There is plenty of laughter to cover up the tears and the pain. Tomorrow, Iliana goes back to the hospital for treatment. And even though we will spend Thanksgiving in a place we have to come to dread, we will be thankful for the people around us, and the family who are always there for us.

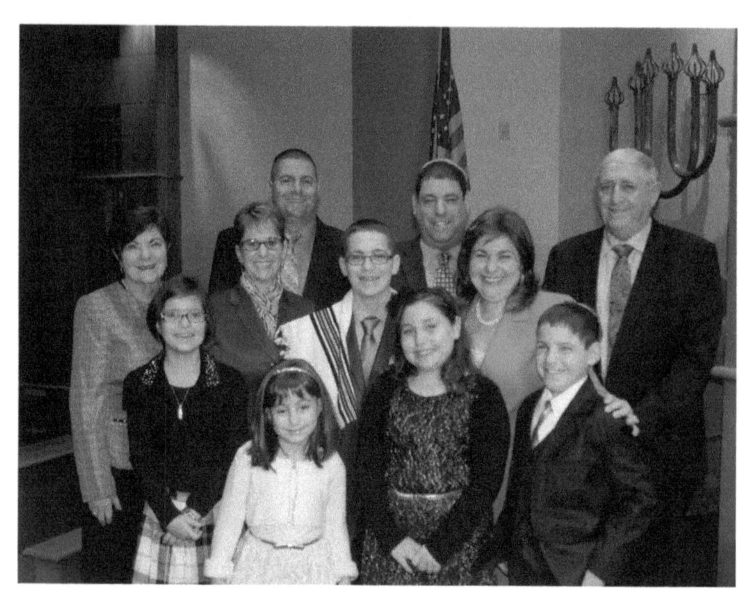

Ezra, Josh, Michael, Joan, Marla, Ross, Me, Sydnee, Iliana, Sarah & Ithan at Ross's Bar Mitzvah.

15

Benefit at Coach's Corner

12/4/2015

Once again, I sit at my computer and write with so many emotions and thoughts in my head. So much has happened this past week, and I feel as though I have touched every realm of the emotional spectrum.

First, we spent Thanksgiving in the hospital. This is one of my favorite holidays. What could have been a tough day ended up being a lot of fun thanks to the wonderful nurses in the hospital. A very generous family sent us food from Magnolias and I got to look around the room at my beautiful family and truly be thankful for what I have. It is okay to be here, because we get to spend it together. We got to be thankful, like many other families in the country. Our location might not have been as glamorous as most, but we were still a "normal" family eating dinner together — a person couldn't ask for much more.

I then received the most wonderful, beautiful gift. Videos and pictures and notes from years of my life. The people who had helped to shape my life took time to remind me that I too had an impact on them (good or bad:)). Thank you, Mechal and Chaim for reminding me how important the past is and how much it impacts the future.

Finally, today NBC did a story talking about the fundraiser tomorrow. Now everyone knows what I have always known, how terrific our community is. I can't even imagine the countless hours that have been dedicated to making tomorrow a success. The businesses and individuals who donated to the silent auction and, of course, our dear friends. The amazing group that did this!

How do I express my gratitude to so many different people? How do I ensure that all those generous individuals and families understand the impact they have had on my family and how their support has truly helped us get through daily? I suppose I can't, but I can try. So, thank you. Thank you from the bottom of my heart for not just the financial help but the emotional support. The reminder of the goodness of people in this harsh reality we live in. The knowledge that you can tackle whatever life throws at you when you surround yourself with incredible people.

Tonight, I get to go to sleep with a full heart, and hopefully tomorrow I will be able to personally thank you.

The benefit at Coach's Corner took a lot of work, but unfortunately, the money that would be raised was needed. Our bank account was really starting to get depleted. We knew my parents, in-laws, my brother and family and countless others would help us if need be, but our pride wouldn't allow it. It was hard to remember that this didn't happen to us because of something we did, we were just unlucky. In fact, we had asked both sets of oncologists (mine and Iliana's) what we needed to change so another member of our family wouldn't be so unlucky. Both sets of doctors said, "*This is a one in a million chance.... You should play the lottery.*"

Healthwise I definitely didn't feel like we won the lottery. I had to remember that not only was our family amazing, but so were our friends. In fact, as part of the fundraiser, all the teams in ULYFL donated baskets and money to us. One coach who is an incredible friend to us wrote to the families of his team, "*I am sure that you have received the league email concerning the Rubins, or heard from other parents. They are close friends of ours and a huge part of our life in Purcellville. Their youngest daughter, Iliana, was diagnosed this summer with leukemia and began immediate chemotherapy treatments. She is a spitfire. She will stare you down and not give up an inch of ground when her mind is made up. She was also the one as a Bengal cheerleader to give me a hug on the 50 yard line before games prior to the team running out. Melt your heart kind of hugs. Their son, Ithan, played on that team with several of our current Oarsmen. Always the youngest and smallest whenever I have had him on my teams, but always the one that I knew would grow the most. Mischievous and infectious in his laugh, he has continued to play this season despite everything going on. Their older sister, Sarah, cheers for the Seahawks. She also calls me "Princess." We share a birthday and one year as we shared a cake she told me, "Blow out the candles, Princess!" It stuck. Watching her deal with this, I wonder that even though I am older, I think she has me beat in maturity at times.*

These kids are the product of Josh and Gina. Josh has coached with me for three years in ULYFL and ULLL. The definition of gregarious. The passion and exuberance he has for the kids and watching them develop and succeed is contagious. I know every season is better standing next to him on the sidelines. The glue that holds all this together is Gina. Amazing person. She keeps four kids in line (including Josh). She embodies charity, love, and friendship. You cannot say hi without a hug. She was also diagnosed herself with Non-Hodgkin's Lymphoma six weeks after Iliana's diagnosis. She has begun six months of chemotherapy. Takes your breath away. But when you see her, she wants to know how you and the kids are doing. This is who they are.

The reason I write this is to put a face on the family. The Rubins are part of what makes ULYFL and Purcellville so great. Genuine caring people. The kind you cannot wait to see at Fireman's Field. As you know, the league has started a fund for them and would like to have all teams make a donation towards the fundraiser. Some teams have done gift baskets, some are taking donations.

The Oarsmen have elected to contribute the money collected for coaches gifts as a sign of solidarity with Josh. I told the other coaches I think we can get by without another gift card to Coaches Corner or Dick's. Not trying to badger anyone, but thought it would be a nice gesture from the other coaches in the league. I apologize if it is out of line."

12/7/2015

For those of you who know Iliana, this little story won't surprise you. To those who don't, here is a taste of this amazing little diva:

An unbelievable family bought the American girl doll basket and gave it to Iliana. She has not stopped playing with it since Saturday. Thank you so much for putting that beautiful smile on her face. Now the conversation between her and Josh:

Iliana: Daddy, what would you like from the bakery?

Josh: I want the ipad.

Iliana: That is not for sale. What do you want to eat?

Josh: I want the ipad. This is poor customer service.
Iliana: Give me back my money. You are no longer a customer!!
Watch out world, Iliana is back!!

12/7/2015

We all have those days that we know we will never forget. The days that you remember your emotions, how you felt, who was there. December 5th is one of those days for me. It is the day that when all this is past us and Iliana and I look back — we will forget the pain of the needles, the anxiety of the spinal tap, the side effects of the chemo. But we will remember when the people we love and the community we cherish just anticipated our needs. You were there when we needed emotional support, to ensure that Sarah and Ithan didn't feel neglected. You knew how much it would help to provide us a meal so that it was one less thing to worry about. And you knew that as much as we try to escape the reality of situations, they exist. Even though getting healthy is our number one priority, we still have financial obligations. And you knew that — you understood the medical bills and the loss of pay.

Thank you, Coach's Corner, for truly emulating what Purcellville is about. Our local "Cheers" where everyone does know your name. Where you walk in on a cold day and warm up not only from the aroma of delicious food, but also the warmth of the atmosphere — the smiles of the waiters/waitresses and the embrace of family that starts with the incredible individuals who own Coach's.

And to the Purcellville community and the ones that surround it, ULYFL and our sports' family — we have always loved being a part of you. You opened your arms and embraced us with the most unbelievable, largest, tightest hug. You reminded us of why growing up in a small town is so precious and why we chose to raise our children here. That the school is not just a place to educate our children, but also a second home and support system. Thank you for teaching my children that the fields are not just to understand competition, but also to learn about teamwork and cherish community.

And, to our dear families and friends that were and are there for us; who put in all their time and effort to make the fundraiser a success. I can't even begin to list everyone for fear of leaving someone out. You know who you are. Thank you for doing this for us — for turning a scary, hard time into a beautiful reality. For making Iliana feel like a princess and giving us such an incredible day. For taking time from your family to help ours. You tell me not to thank you; but how can I not. You have taught our children the true meaning of friendship, what it means to give all yourself to help a friend. When I see you, I will try to refrain from thanking you. :) But at least let me promise you this. Josh and I will try to always be the friend you deserve. We will always be there to support and love you and in fifty years will still be in Coach's Corner laughing and probably disturbed by our husbands' comments. And when you need a ride or shoulder to cry on, I will be here. Maybe you can meet me at Coach's; I will buy you a beer.

The event raised twenty-five thousand dollars. So many people who own businesses donated via the fundraiser and Sip & Shop. At the Sip & Shop, there were vendors from Silipada, Wildtree, Mary Kay, Scentsy, Thirty-one, EVER Skincare, KEEP jewelry, Stella & Dot, Usborne books, Jamberry, Doterra, Tupperware and Lululemon. Valley Energy gave us free gas for the year and gave us money back. Western Loudoun Basketball, Upper Loudoun Baseball — all rec sports' leagues donated money to us. I could not believe the sheer amount of support we received. The money was used to pay the mortgage, medical bills, and other bills. Without it, I don't know what we would have done. I think we might have had to move. A lot of our friends wanted us to use it for fun but reality dictated we had to use it for necessities. I know I mentioned this a lot, but we were so lucky that our friends did this for us. Without their support, our lives might have been devoid of cheer, compassion and love.

16
Chemotoxicity

1/7/2016

From Josh: It has been a while since we have posted anything on this page so we apologize for not keeping you up to speed with what has been going on.

Let's start with Iliana:

Iliana continues to be doing well with her treatments. She started her latest phase of treatment last Wednesday with a completely new chemotherapy and a spinal tap. So far, she has taken this very well. She is on steroids this month, which will hopefully help her gain a little more weight, but the good news is that she isn't losing any. Her hair has come back pretty quickly, but unfortunately with the chemo that she is on now, it will likely go away again. Good thing is that from a moral perspective, Iliana has seen that her hair will come back and come back quickly so she is not concerned. She is in great spirits and bouncing off the walls and has even been able to see her best friend, Ryleigh, a few times over the past week, which has made her days. Hopefully, Iliana will continue on this path as she is scheduled to end her treatment towards the end of March and will go onto a maintenance schedule for the following two years, which will be much less invasive and intense.

Regarding Gina:

Reason we have been quite delayed in posting any update is because we ran into a little setback with Gina. A few weeks back, Gina had a negative reaction to one of the chemotherapy treatments she was on. It is called chemotoxicity and this particular side effect impacts the back of the brain that deals with speech and balance. It has really impaired her ability to walk and speak clearly. She was in the hospital for eleven days and was discharged right before Christmas. Unfortunately, this side effect really has hit her hard and up until this past weekend, progress was at a snail's pace. Fortunately, over this past weekend, Gina made a turn for the best. She is still not one hundred percent back to her normal self, but has been able to speak a lot better and has been able to walk around on her own with very little balance issues. This toxicity side effect should completely wear off and Gina should be back to normal, but we are not one hundred percent sure how long it will take. It is quite frustrating to her because, as you all know, Gina is very independent and hasn't been able to be for the past three weeks. As long as there are signs of progress, we are all happy. Yesterday, Gina had her second PET scan to determine if there was identifiable cancer throughout her body that the original PET scan showed back in September. Today we went to her oncologist for a follow-up appointment (first since she was discharged from the hospital) so that we can find out what the next steps are with regards to her treatment and to find out the results of the scan. The doctor said that he is going to suspend her treatment so she can continue to recover and that she will start back up with a different chemotherapy regimen in about one and a half weeks assuming she has recovered. The bad news is that this will extend her treatments into March. Fortunately, this bad news seemed to be immediately forgotten after her doctor gave us the news that GINA IS CANCER FREE!!!!! Her PET Scan was completely normal and there were no signs of cancer. What an absolute relief! Regardless of these results, Gina will continue to get chemo as this is part of the regimen to ensure that she remains cancer free going forward. So now both Gina and Iliana are technically cancer free and are just finishing up the remainder of their treatments as part of their plan. Hopefully things will continue on this path and we can continue to provide good news on this page.

This all said, I want to personally thank our family and friends (near and far) who have kept us in their thoughts and prayers. It has been absolutely overwhelming the amount of support we have received; from the house cleanings, babysitting for the kids while I was at the hospital with Gina, lawn service, the dinners that are provided, carpools for the other kids, piano lessons for Iliana, dog food delivery, Costco and grocery store runs, extremely successful fundraisers managed by our wonderful friends and many other things that have been done that have helped us out in so many ways. You all have been a critical piece to me personally getting through this and I know I speak to the feelings of the rest of my family. You have been willing to basically drop what you were doing to immediately help us out without hesitation or question. I hope that we will never have to repay you as I do not want anyone to have to go through this, but please know that the Rubins will forever be indebted to you and love you all and will have your backs if the need ever arises.

Until next update..... F#K CANCER!!!*

I have not spoken much about work. No question, my job has been wonderful to me. When I found out Iliana had cancer, I was able to work from the hospital or at home to be with Iliana. When I learned about my cancer, they insisted I work exclusively from home. This would stop extra germs from infecting Iliana or myself.

I didn't think I was experiencing any side effects from the chemo but apparently I was. I was forgetting a lot and making uncharacteristic mistakes. Fortunately, my boss was able to catch them, but when he pointed them out, I was surprised as I didn't think I made them. Over time, I learned I had chemo brain. I always thought that chemo brain was just an excuse, but admittedly I was floored in reference to all the mistakes I was making. Because of this, I spoke to my boss about going out on short-term disability at the end of the year. Little did I know that I would end up having to take it earlier.

Our friends, the Owens, always host extraordinary Christmas parties. I will always remember that night (Saturday, December 12, 2015), I started feeling dizzy. I was excited for the party but I felt so ill that I told Josh to go alone. He was hesitant to leave me but I insisted. The next morning, I was still dizzy, so we called the oncologist on call. He didn't seem worried, but he advised us to go to Loudoun Hospital just to be safe. The kids came out of their rooms to ask how I was. Josh told them to go downstairs into the playroom. He didn't know how I would do going down the stairs and he didn't want to scare them. Sarah, being the nosy one, peeked out and saw me fall down a few stairs. Luckily, Josh was there to catch me and he steadied me down the rest of the stairs. Ithan called Mindy and asked her to please come over. She and Ronnie dropped everything and came. They watched the kids, along with my parents, and Josh drove me to the ER. The doctors at the ER thought maybe it was vertigo. They kept me overnight in the observation ward. The ward was set up so it looked like ER rooms, and I wasn't actually "admitted" but I was being monitored. At one point, I needed to go to the bathroom. I carefully walked to the bathroom but once in the bathroom, I couldn't keep my balance. I fell down and the nurses came rushing in and assisted me back to my bed. After making sure that I hadn't injured myself, they left me to try to sleep through the remainder of the night. The next day, I attempted to open my eyes but I couldn't. I heard Josh come in and I tried to whisper to him that I couldn't open my eyes. My words came out slurred. I was so scared, and I didn't know what was happening. I could be blind, not be able to speak clearly, and who knows what else. The fear of the unknown once again gripped me. What if I never saw Sarah's green eyes anymore, Ithan play baseball, or Iliana's brown hair once it grew back. I would never see what beautiful women my girls grew into or how handsome my son was.

I was admitted into the hospital. Even though the hospital is void of pleasure (especially for us), I was placed in a big corner room with its own two door entrance. The room itself had a comfy recliner, a sitting bench which lined the window, and a huge bathroom. This wasn't a castle but I felt like a queen.

I heard the doctor come in to check on me. I tried to explain that I couldn't open my eyes and he could hear my inability to speak. I don't think the doctors knew at the time what was wrong with me. I then heard Ezra and Marla come visit, and even though I felt my eyes moving back and forth, I couldn't open them. It was Sunday and I remember wanting to watch the Redskins play. I was annoyed because I couldn't watch something as simple as a football game. Thinking back about it as I write this it seems silly, but that must have been my way of expressing my frustration at not being able to see and not understanding what was happening.

Fortunately, after a few days the medicated eye drops the doctor put in my eyes worked and I was able to open them. I was still struggling with eating and talking. It was easier to not eat and be hungry than it was to lift a fork to my mouth. I remember my mother was coming to relieve Josh as he had to do something. My mother asked me what I wanted to eat; I felt like pizza. She brought me some type of gourmet slice but I ended up only taking a few bites as aligning my mouth to the food was extremely difficult. During my stay in the hospital, I lived on Coke.

My "vacation" in the hospital was a humbling and mortifying experience. I had to call the nurse every time I went to the bathroom as I went from being dizzy to having an extremely hard time walking. I required help to move so a person always had to be nearby. As a 39-year-old woman, I needed help cleaning myself, so the nurse bathed me. I had to undress in front of her, which didn't phase her but I was mortified! What a production an everyday event became for me. I had to call the nurse, a chair had to be placed in the shower so I could sit, my hair was shampooed and my body cleaned, all with someone else's help. After eleven days at my new home, I was finally released but with a new toy — a wheelchair! This was insane; my new reality was awful! I needed help going to and from the bathroom, and someone was always home with me just in case I fell. I couldn't drive, cook — anything! I had lost all my independence.

My oncologist insisted on a follow-up. Josh had to drive me to the doctor's office and wheel me into the waiting room. Hearing I had cancer was horrible, but not having any independence without knowing what the future holds was terrible and scary!

Something that saved my life (chemo) also was causing such havoc. Of course, I am grateful that chemo was chasing the cancer away, but how could I be thankful when the same poison was causing me such unbelievable strain and anguish.

17

Iliana is Back at School

Inspiration
3/14/2016

It has been a while since I posted, which is a good thing. It means we are doing okay. :). I am posting now for a few reasons.

First, to let you know that we are doing well!! My last week of treatment is next week!! We can see the light; we are both so close!!! Iliana is her amazing diva self. She has so much energy, it's impossible to keep up with her.

Inspiration — I have heard that word so much in the past few months. It is a word that has brought tears to my eyes so many different times. Sarah was asked to write an "inspiration" piece at school and she wrote about Iliana. Her words were so beautiful, I had to control my tears. But she is correct! Iliana is an inspiration. She doesn't argue about not being able to go anywhere. She takes her chemo like a champ!! She doesn't cry. She is always in a great mood, no matter what! She is my inspiration!! How can I be upset if she is so happy? How can I not have a stiff upper lip if she looks at every day as though it is another great day? She makes me stronger and happier, her attitude is so uplifting.

Yesterday, we went to Ithan's team party as a family. This is the first time in a long time. To watch Iliana run around like a normal little girl was the most unbelievable thing!! It has been a while since she has been able to behave like that and it made her night. Ithan's coach also said some words about each boy. He used the word inspiration. He was thankful to have had Ithan on his team, and was grateful that he got to be a part of our journey. He said "we inspired him!!" His words brought tears to my eyes, as we weren't easy to have on the team yet he was grateful to us.

And finally, today my kids got the surprise of their life!! The Harlem Globetrotters came to visit Iliana's clinic. They were amazing!!! They took pictures with everyone and truly brightened the whole place up! Then we got tickets to their game on Saturday. The kids are soooooooo excited! (Thank you to Chaim and Mechal who made this possible).

These past few months have brought so much pain into our house. But there has also been so much kindness and laughter and yes, inspiration. Look at what inspires you. When you kiss your kids, look into their innocent eyes. Be inspired by them; they have so much goodness to give. When you hug them, hug them tight because they love you no matter what! I am inspired when I look around Iliana's clinic and see the smiles on the kids faces even though they have suffered more than we can imagine. I am inspired by how Sarah and Ithan have responded to all that has happened. And I am inspired by organizations like the Globetrotters who brighten up what could be a dreary day.

May you find your inspiration.

4/27/2016

It is amazing how your perspective changes due to the path you take. The kids were eating breakfast and started talking about what they would wish for if they had three wishes. Ithan wants to be the Nat's batboy and meet Stephen Curry. Most little girls would wish to be a princess, but Iliana just wanted to be in maintenance and spend the day at her best friend's house. Today her wish came true because she started maintenance and she might go to her best buddy's house this weekend as well!

Normally, we all start school around September, send our children to football, soccer, piano, etc., and so on and so forth. We try to figure out how to do it all — how can we get everything done and ensure that our kids still get a healthy meal, their homework done, and still get a good night's sleep? Unfortunately, this wasn't what we had to worry about this past school year. Instead, we had to figure out who stayed in the hospital with Iliana, who would take Ithan and Sarah to practice, how to ensure that Sarah and Ithan were okay — and that they knew life would be all right. The good news is that life is good — Iliana starts school on Monday!!! It is her first day of not only school but hopefully what will become her normal life again.

That, of course, is the best news possible. But fortunately, so much else has happened. I am done with my treatments. My final PET scan showed that I was cancer free. Even though I still have remnants of the chemotoxicity, I still got to see Ithan score his first soccer goal, see Sarah do amazing things in her first year of middle school, enjoy all the great news about my niece and nephew, and celebrate Iliana's road to health, really get to experience how amazing she truly is. I also got to once again see how truly wonderful my community is:

The KWC talent show, run by the beautiful Rosie Bundick, was dedicated to Iliana and me. Two of Sarah's buddies came back to the school and choreographed a gorgeous ballet to "the sun will come out tomorrow." The terrific kids of KWC sang that song to Iliana and me while bringing us flowers. I, of course, was crying, but Iliana had the most beautiful smile on her face. Thank you for that special evening. It meant so much to us, it will never be forgotten.

I have probably cried more these past few weeks then I have these past few months. Thankfully, these are tears of joy. I cried when we went to Baltimore as a family. I am sure I will cry when Iliana eats her first strawberry in months or goes back to school, jumps out the car to hang at her best friend's house, or goes on her first field trip with her class. I have so much to be thankful for, it will take me months to tell you about it. I am thankful that I got to sit around the Seder table on Passover with my whole family (Josh would have skipped it; in fact, if you have a good reason to save him next year, he will be forever grateful. :)), help my mom get ready for the holiday (my feet hurt but I wouldn't change my time with her for anything), my friend Tracy dedicating her LLS woman of the year campaign to us, my amazing children, and without a doubt, Josh. He has been through so much but he hasn't complained once! He had to drop me off at the hospital for my first treatments and leave me. He felt bad because he had to go home and do what — take care of Iliana! He switched between being at home and sitting in the hospital with me when I got chemotoxicity. And he managed to still get the kids to practice. He has done so much, I don't know how he has stayed so sane (well,sane for Josh) and he has been one of the main reasons I have been able to smile.

And to end, once again I thank you for being there for me and my family. All of you — my parents, in-laws, my brother, his family and our friends. Together we will celebrate the excitement that I know this year will bring. And as those terrific angels of

KWC sang, "the sun will come out tomorrow" or in our case it will continue to come out.

With love and gratitude

My excuse just went to school :) 5/2/2016

The house is so quiet, way too quiet! I was looking forward to going back to work, but now I am really looking forward to it. (I think it's because I have no excuse not to clean out my closet. :). I have plenty to do, just no motivation to do it. I think part of my problem is that I am a little worried, or maybe because I have no one to cuddle. Don't get me wrong, this is great!! Iliana's first day of school!! I can't believe it. We are slowly going back to normal. She got to spend time at her best buddy's house this weekend and spend time with her best buddy at school as well!!

And this morning — what a welcome she had. First, we took her first day picture with her friends who specifically came early for her. Thank you so much for doing that. She didn't stop smiling! Then she was welcomed with a big hug in her class. I have always loved our school, but this year, wow!!! They have been so good to us, and even though having her back adds some more work for the school, they are so excited to have her return!!

I have to admit, I tried so hard not to cry. I was good, only a few tears. It was hard but I didn't want her class to think I was crazy. :) As I write this, this is all still so surreal to me. I still can't believe any of this has occurred. I think I am going to wake up from a bad dream with long flowing hair and remember that I need to get dinner ready so that we can get to practice and bed on time. But I am awake. This actually happened, but it is okay, because we are now celebrating, enjoying and loving our life.

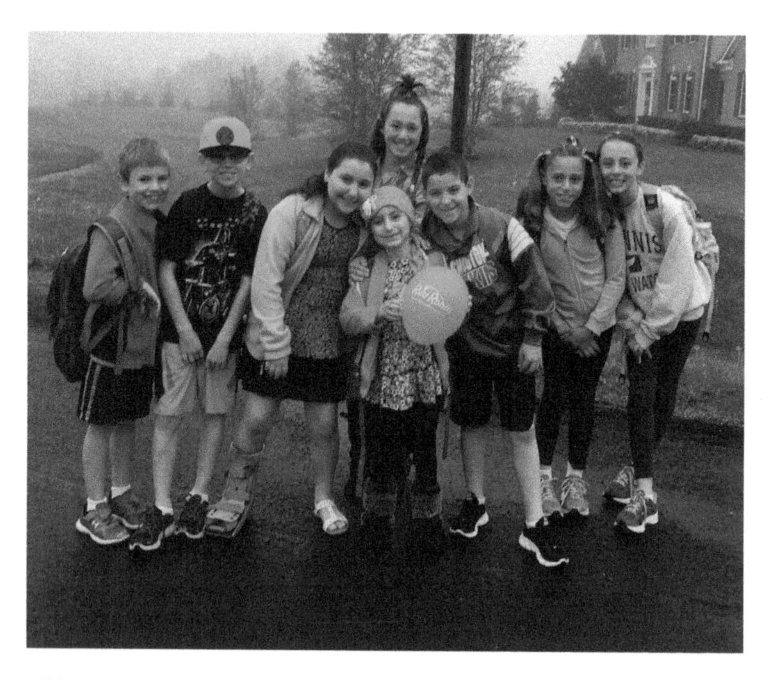

Iliana and some of her neighbor friends on her first day back at school.

I guess I should get to my closet. Nah!! I think I will count down the hours till school is out.

9/22/2016

I can't believe that it is football season again!! Even though this year I get to sit on the sideline and cheer for the Seahawks (Sarah is helping assist the cheerleaders) and the Oursman (Josh is an assistant coach), I feel like every team has some children that I adore. It makes me realize that in a few years I will really be sitting on the sideline with no blood relatives to cheer for. But no matter what, whether I have immediate family on the field or not, I will always be cheering because ULYFL is part of my family. I have always enjoyed watching our kids play on the field, but it is what they learn off the field that I will always cherish.

As most of you know, last year was tough, but the families that make up ULYFL were there for us. You taught us generosity, kindness, and camaraderie. You made our year so much easier. You always had a hug for me, well wishes for us, were ready to drive Sarah and Ithan, and most of all, made Iliana feel like a queen. No matter where life takes me, I will never forget what my small town's football league did. Thank you so much for always being there. Thank you for teaching my kids skills and life's lessons, and thank you for your friendship. I will always remember what you did for my family. Make sure you treasure every moment for they only last a while, but if you are as lucky as me, you will be surrounded by precious people who make these cherished moments. Go ULYFL!!

Your lifelong fan

Josh and Ithan have always loved hockey. We have always cheered for the Washington Capitals because they were Josh's and Ithan's favorite team, but I never really cared for the sport as much as football. That all changed for not only me, but for Iliana as well when we were invited to the hockey fights cancer event that the Caps hosted locally. The Caps Fight Cancer event was so heartwarming. First, the whole family was invited to take part in a Washington Capitals practice session at the Kettler Iceplex. Everyone got to watch the practice, and afterwards, were invited onto the ice to spend time with the players and skated with the player they were matched up with. Iliana was matched up with Zach Sanford. Even though he was a rookie at the time, he was very compassionate toward Iliana, and an onlooker would have thought him a veteran player. Sarah ended up skating with Tom Wilson since his buddy had to leave early. Alex Ovechkin was partnered with a child born with a few deformities who then got cancer. This young man could ice skate so quickly, he was like a cheetah on ice, and it was hard to tell he was sick. Ovechkin gave him his popular yellow shoelaces and his hockey stick. Even though these hockey players are tough men, they will tell you they look up to these young fighters.

The next part of the event was the game at Capital One Arena the following day. During pregame, Zach wore Iliana's last name in place of his own on his purple Caps Fight Cancer practice jersey. All of the players wore jerseys representing a child who was fighting cancer, and it was amazing to see. Even more amazing was that the players took the time to meet and get to know the child and their families. During this special game, there was an online auction going on, selling much of the game worn Caps Fight Cancer gear, and I am proud to say that Zach's practice jersey with Iliana's name on it and hockey stick are now prominently displayed in our house.

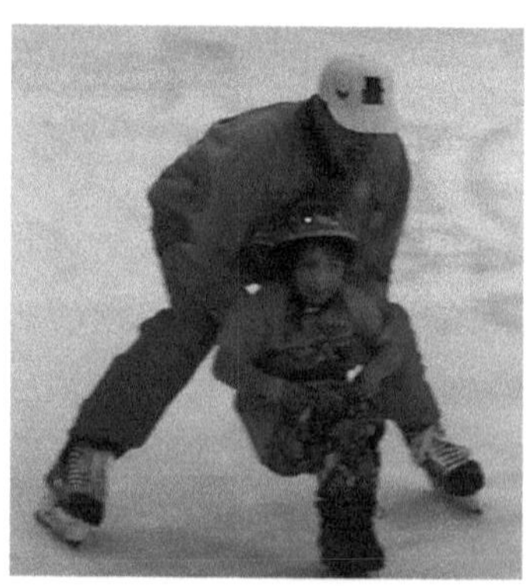

Zach and Iliana.

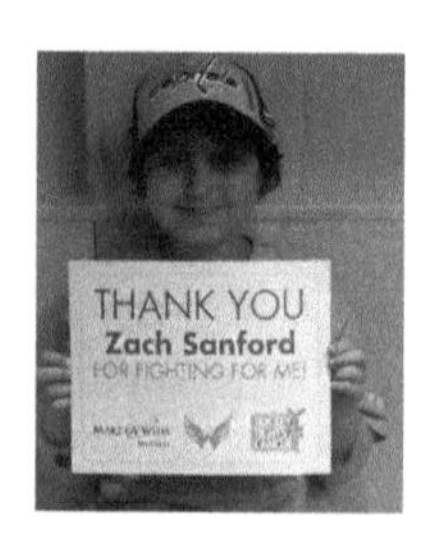

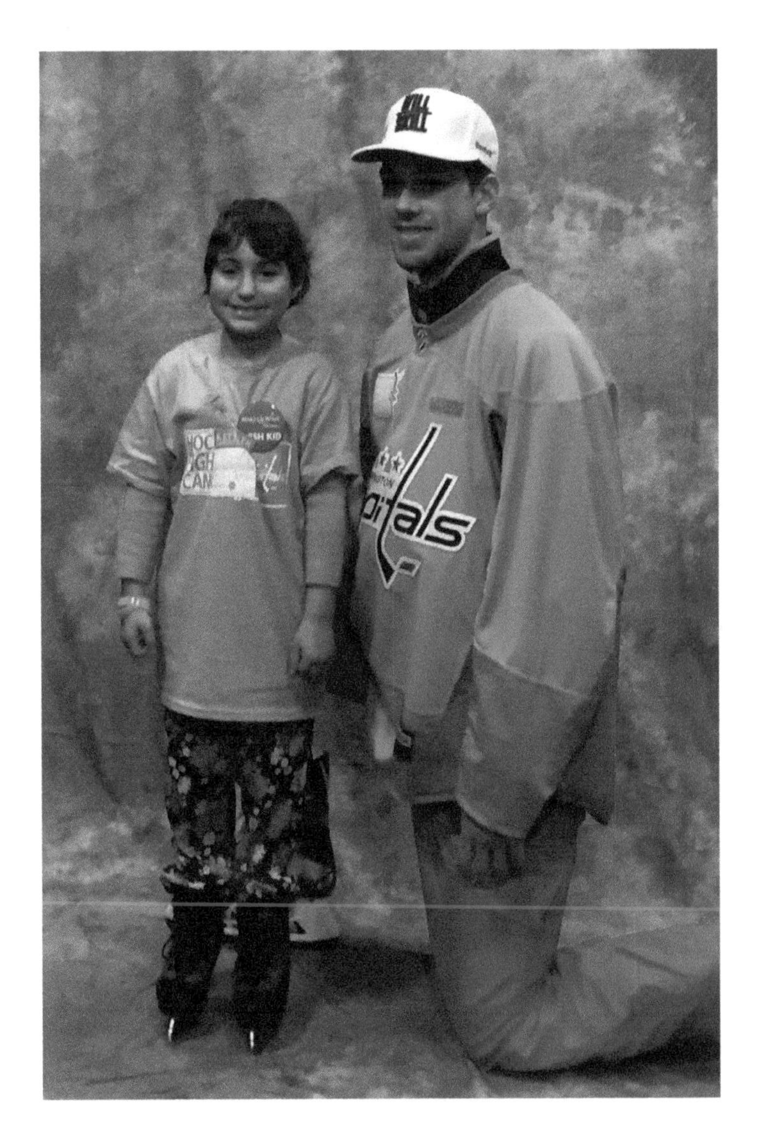

After the game, Iliana and the rest of the children fighting cancer were invited into the locker room to be a part of the post game celebration of the Capital's win. We will never forget this experience and Zach will always be a friend, even though he is no longer on the Washington Capitals.

12/19/2016

It has been a while since I have written and it will hopefully be a while before I write again. A lot has happened — mainly good and a little bad. I will start with the bad, which fortunately ended up okay. :) During Iliana's maintenance, there were a couple weeks where her numbers were low. We were told that this could happen for a couple reasons — too much chemo for her body or a relapse.

That word "relapse" made me think of the worst week of my life. The week we were told Iliana had leukemia — the emotional roller coaster was a nightmare. Fortunately, it was the former but those few days I was a wreck.

Luckily, the rest of this post is good. :) I will never be grateful that I got cancer and especially that Iliana got cancer, but I am thankful for the good I got to see and the people I met. There is a saying, "It's during tough times that you know who your real friends are." I can honestly say that I did find out — that everyone I called my friend was there for my family and I was lucky enough to make and meet more. The organizations and people who were there for us were amazing! I will highlight just a few. Our new and gorgeous friend — Tracy Robinson. After battling and thankfully winning her own fight, she was determined to turn her hard journey into finding a way to make it easier for others. She raised over one hundred thousand dollars dollars for the Leukemia & Lymphoma Society in just ten weeks. She dedicated her fight to Iliana and me and is now our hairdresser. :) We love how she does our hair, but even more we are better because she is in our life.

We also got to meet Jay Coakley, the founder of Ellie's Hats. He is such a terrific person and we are so much better for knowing him.

Then we were honored to become part of the Make-a-Wish family. We were invited to join the Washington Capitals for their Caps Fight Cancer weekend. I don't know much about hockey, but I am now infatuated with the Capitals. :) We got to meet amazing people like T.J Oshie, who said you skate your whole life but you don't know that in your future you get to impact other lives. He is such an unbelievable person! And we were lucky enough to be matched up with Zach Sanford (#82). He is a rookie and not a household name (yet) but one of the sweetest guys you will ever meet. He went out of his way for us, and we are so lucky that he is part of our life. (He is so quiet, so you can just imagine how ironic that he was matched up with our loud, chaotic family.) I hope that we can bring him joy like he has brought us.

I cannot believe 2016 is almost over! No question the second half of 2015 was awful and 2016 was better but not great. But we are here and we are ready to write our next chapter. It will be terrific. In fact, we have our first entry — hopefully Iliana's last treatment is in October! Thank you to everyone for being there for us, for making our rollercoaster ride a bit smoother and for allowing us to know that great people do exist in this world. Thank you for being friends that are there for us no matter what. I was given a plaque with a beautiful saying, "When it hurts to look back and you're afraid to look ahead, look beside you and there will be your friends."

To all our friends, Happy New Year and thank you for being part of our next chapter.

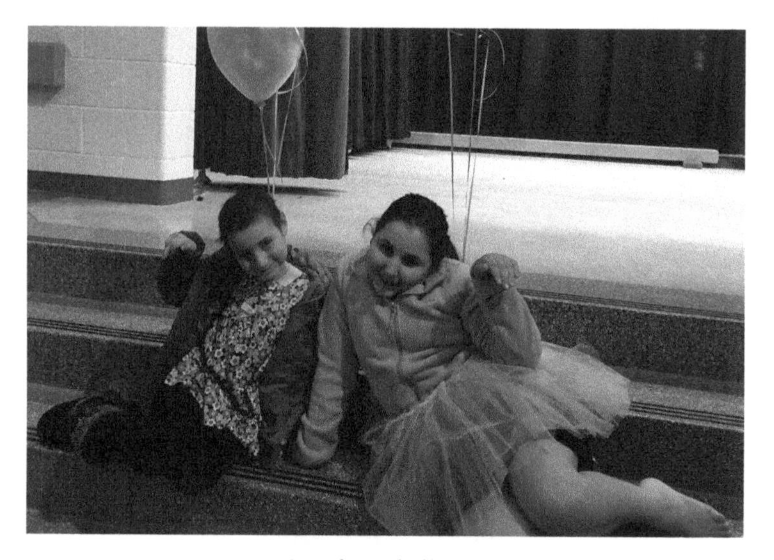

Sarah and Iliana.

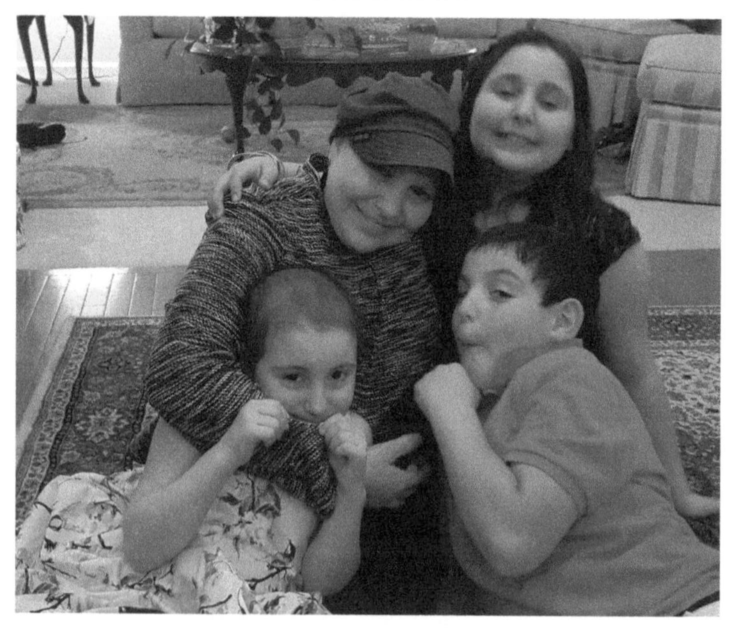

Kids and Gina at Nona's House.

Part Three
Girls Can Fight

18

We are Done!

In February of 2017, we were granted a Make-a-Wish trip on a Disney cruise. It was an all-inclusive trip. It even included a "wish" party with a catered lunch before we left. We invited our family and friends to our house for the party. After the party, we rode to Reagan Airport in a limousine, flew to Orlando and boarded the beautiful Disney Wonder.

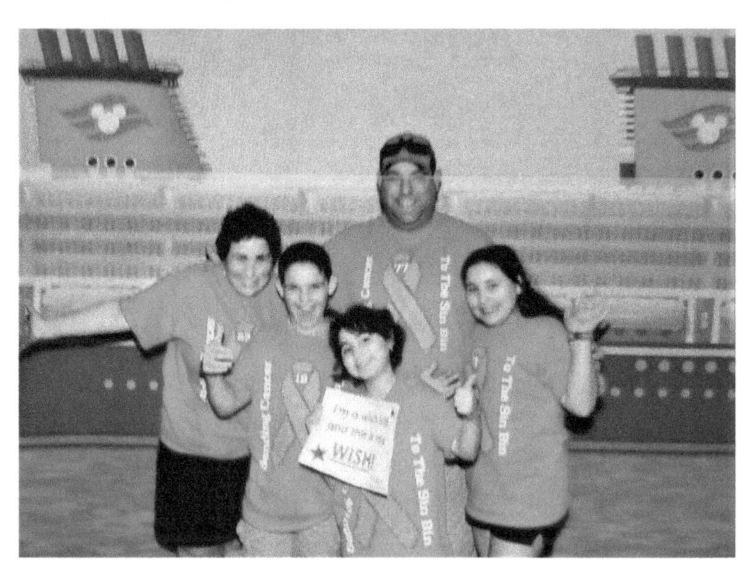

We wore t-shirts, compliments of CustomInk, that we had the opportunity to design for the trip. Overall, it was an amazing cruise; we were treated like royalty. Our room was fitted with a queen size bed and three beds that turned into comfortable sofas during the day. We got special treats throughout the cruise; Disney along with the Make-a-Wish organization really knows how to make a miserable time somewhat enjoyable. If nothing else, they know how to take your mind off the suffering.

10/10/2017

It has been a bittersweet few months. I say "bitter" for a few reasons but I will mention one. On August 21, we had to say goodbye to our twelve-year-old chocolate lab, Annie. She died of (something this house is all too familiar with) cancer. She snuggled with Iliana and I while we had to endure our treatments and was always by our side. It is thought that animals know when we are suffering and I believe that to be true. For all you naysayers out there — yes, even Baxter. He is always good for a laugh or kiss.

I say "sweet" because tomorrow is Iliana's last treatment of chemo! Her final day of all chemo pills is October 28th! No more worrying when she ate last or if she took her medicine. The doctor said her port can come out when she has a few months in a row of good numbers.

I have thanked a lot of amazing people in my posts except for one phenomenal little girl, Iliana's BFF, Ryleigh. She has been with Iliana since day one. What amazes me most about her is that she never shuddered at Iliana. Even when Iliana had the feeding tube or no hair, Ryleigh only cared that she got to see Iliana! I am sure her wonderful family helped her by preparing her, but there is no question that she helped Iliana have so much strength. My usual weekend wake-up call is, "Can Ryleigh come over?" (Baxter will kill me if I don't give a shout-out to Ryleigh's dad, Mike — Baxter's BFF) It is such a good feeling that Iliana feels the same love and strength from her friends that I have gotten.

We are not one hundred percent sure of what the next year will bring but at least we see the light at the end of the tunnel. Thank you again, friends and family, new and old, for helping us get through these tough past few years. And even though I know that the future might not be easy (the residual effects from chemo can cause a lot of side effects), at least we can look the future in its eye and say, "Cancer came for us, but we won!" (Phrase coined by Sarah Rubin).

10/11/2017

We are finally done with chemo. When we started this tough journey, we never thought this day would ever come. Iliana got to ring the "I am done with chemo" bell. We happily hugged everyone goodbye and skipped out of the clinic.

Unfortunately, our next stop was the hospital. Even though our tough and grueling journey is slowing down, our friends' travels are just beginning for they just found out their son has leukemia. Without a doubt, this will be the hardest road they will have to venture down. But I did learn that it is very important to accept everyone's help. I like to do things myself, but it truly is a blessing in disguise for not only your family but also for those who are reaching out.

The first week was a roller coaster of emotions and I didn't want to talk to anyone. I eventually learned that it was important to use all the resources that were available and this was a road not to travel alone. Please let us help in anyway we can —for us at least we will be able to use what we had to learn to help an awesome family. Think of it as you allowing us to give back. We got so much from our amazing community, friends and family. It is our turn to be there now; please allow us to do this. It doesn't seem like it now, but this too will pass and even in your darkest hour, we will be there for you, and soon your precious child will be ringing that wonderful bell too.

10/28/2017

AND WE ARE DONE!!! October 11th was Iliana's last treatment and today was her last chemo pill hopefully forever. When this all started at the end of July 2015, it seemed like this day would never come. But we did it!! She still has to endure another surgery when her port comes out and more shots when she has to get her immunizations again. But at least she doesn't have to wait 3 hours to eat anymore and soon she can eat whatever she wants. (Hopefully her taste buds come back; they can change because of chemo.) She is very excited to eat lox again (even though your salmon cream cheese, Ezra Elkon, is close, it is not lox.) And watch out, Oma and Zeida, because she wants Biltong!

Our lives will never be the same, but at least we can live it. Thank you to everyone who has been there for us. I am lucky enough to say that I can't list everybody because I would be here until tomorrow night. You know who you are and always know, you will forever be engraved in my heart.

With love and gratitude

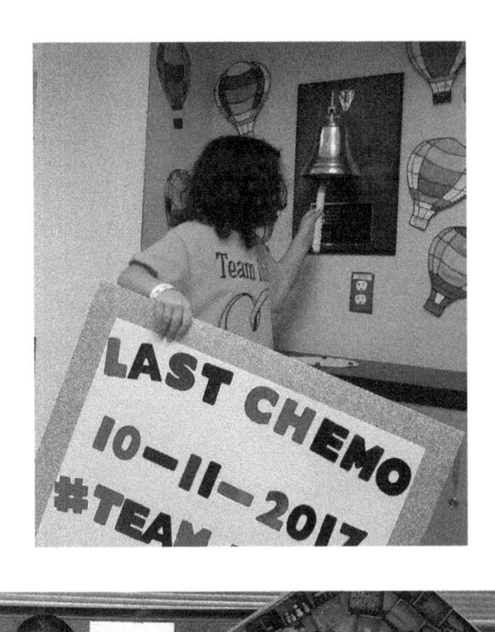
LAST CHEMO

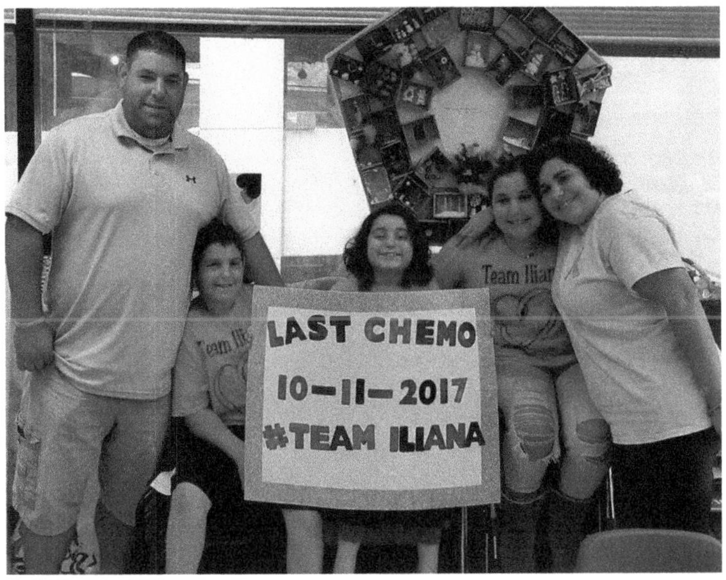
LAST CHEMO
10-11-2017
#TEAM ILIANA

Part Four

Thunder Keeps Rolling: Life After Cancer

19

Cancer Keeps on Giving

1/6/2018

It has been over two years since our amazing fundraiser hosted by Tanya Owens and Brandy Payne at our very own Coach's Corner Grill. Not to mention the scores of people who helped make our fundraiser an amazing success and Danielle Kabban who held the Sip and Shop at her house. There, too, were scores of vendors who gave their proceeds to us. I will never forget this, as the money raised helped us a tremendous amount. We hope to use the money for other families who are suffering and are not as lucky as we are to have such tremendous support. (We have had to use some of it to pay some bills, but as soon as I find a full-time job, we hope to be able to replenish it).

I take for granted that family is always there, because I am happy to say, mine is. I forget that a lot of people suffer without anyone to comfort them or make them laugh. I still suffer from some of the effects of chemo as I definitely have my days where I remember how I used to be. My career was moving quickly in an upward trajectory and even though Ithan beat me, I loved playing basketball with him. I was not scared to dance with my girls and I loved to talk and hang out with my friends. These moments,

I know I am hard to be around, but when I turn, everyone is still there for me. Watch out world, because soon I will be back!

I am lucky to say that our friends are still around. In fact, I have had the opportunity to be closer to some of them. Even though I am done, there is a saying that cancer keeps on giving. And even though this phrase is meant in a derogatory manner, there are some good and some amazing moments that have come out of this horrible disease. One such moment happened last night. Woodgrove hosted Valley in basketball for the cancer night. Each player wore the last name of the cancer survivor or fighter they played for and gave them a beautiful flower. Matthew Thomas played for me.

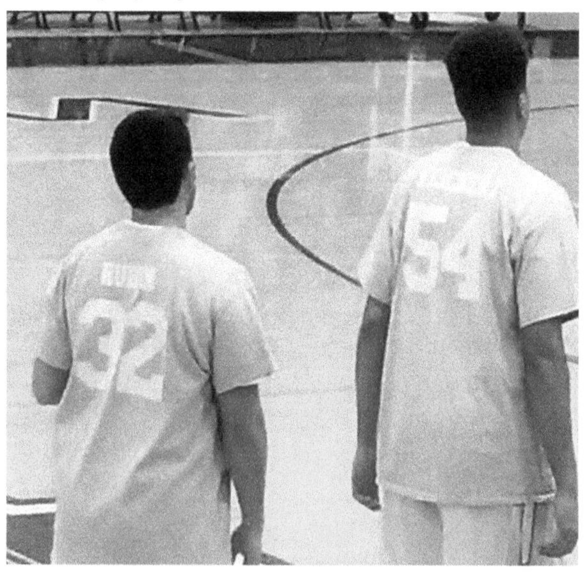

Matthew Thomas playing for me in the Woodgrove versus Loudoun Valley cancer game.

I don't think he knows what it means to me that such a wonderful young man wore my last name on his back. I don't have a daughter his age, and that is why poor Patrick is stuck with me. As his mom and I were joking, at Patrick's wedding, when it is asked, "Does anyone object to this wedding?", if it is not to one of my girls — I will.

2017 ended with a bang. I can't say it was a terrific year but it ended like no other. Iliana got her port out! Here's to 2018 being the best year for all of us, and may you be as lucky as us to have the greatest family and friends surround you! And don't forget, GIRLS CAN FIGHT! :)

20

Team LoCo on Cancer

In 2018, Sarah was part of team "LoCo on Cancer," an LLS Student of the Year (SOY) team based out of Loudoun County. Her team didn't raise the most money, but the reasons they did it were inspiring. Some did it because they knew someone who had battled cancer, and some did it because they wanted to give back. Sarah did it because, besides having a beautiful heart, she unfortunately had two very close reasons to raise money for this particular charity.

The team put together some amazing fundraising events. One of the most original and memorable one was a toilet that was painted red and had the words "Flush Cancer" on it. The toilet was placed in someone's yard and that person had to pay a "ransom" to have it removed and got to choose the next recipient of the toilet. People were also given the opportunity to pay "insurance" to not have the toilet placed in their yards.

The money the team raised was in honor of Sara Willis. A truly unbelievable child who passed away from cancer before her 18th birthday.

This is what I wrote:

Thank you for all of your generous donations to LoCo on Cancer SOY campaign. Because of your generosity over sixty thousand dollars was raised and a grant in precious Sara Willis' name will be given. You know she is smiling from heaven and dancing as these amazing kids collected over two million dollars dollars for LLS. Some, unfortunately, are connected to cancer because a loved one has/had it or they lost someone because of it. Others are doing it because they want to give back. It doesn't matter why or even what. Unfortunately, my family does what we can for cancer because we understand what it does; someone else might donate their time or money for MS. It doesn't matter what, as long as it's something.

The kids didn't raise the most but they won the community involvement award. I believe this award is given to the team that involves their community the most. I can't tell you what an amazing feeling it was to hear someone exclaim, "Yes, it's my turn to display the toilet!" It was said like it was a rite of passage. Now a lot of people learned what I knew all along — what a great community Purcellville is. Sarah was asked to speak and she did very well. I am also a little biased. :))

Of course, this amazing team was led by Tracy Robinson, who I am happy to say is a very close friend. Josh and I are lucky because we have such amazing parental role models. My kids are lucky because they have such unbelievable external role models. If any of my kids grow up to be anything like Tracy with her generous heart, I will be grateful. She is truly beautiful inside and gorgeous outside!

Thank you, Purcellville, for being the great community you are and thank you, Tracy, for being you and for being a part of our life.

2/4/2019

I had my nine-month checkup with Dr. Spira. My mother came with me. The great news was that everything looked awesome and I was told I wouldn't have to see him for one year. However, I asked him if my speech would ever improve. He, unfortunately, thinks that my speech will stay the same. Only one percent of cancer patients fall in this category. I was this fun-loving, outgoing individual who loved to act, dance, make speeches in public and play basketball. But cancer took that away from me. My career was projecting in a quick upward line. Now, it is propelling down in a quick spiral. I loved interviews, talking on the phone and making people laugh. Cancer changed all that. I am usually a very positive person, but I am starting to feel hopeless. I really want to give up. I wouldn't be a burden on anyone. However, I cannot do that; it's not in my DNA. I told my friend, I really miss me. I had a lot of fixing to do with the old me; however, it was still the old me. The new "me" is too quiet, slurs her words, isn't funny, or in my opinion, fun. I know that a lot of people suffer hardships in their lives. A lot of times they come out in front and are able to become a better person; however, I really feel the opposite with this. Cancer was hard and it sucked, but the after effects are harder for me to handle. I already didn't dance at my daughter's Bat Mitzvah or speak like I would want to. Parties have become hard for me to go to, and going out is an issue for me. My friends went to this pop-up bar and started dancing. I really wanted to join them. The old me would have jumped right in and had a blast. The new "me" was too scared to dance, and I had to leave because otherwise I would have started crying. It is so unfair to my husband who realized I was miserable and had to leave as well.

21

No Confidence

I really feel for Josh, I do. He doesn't know what to do. I am very thankful he tried. He wants me to talk to someone, but I don't think it will help. They can't make me the person I was. They can't have me talk like I used to, walk like I used to, and more importantly, think like I used to. I feel like a totally different person. I used to be so adventurous, and now most things scare me. I believe it is because I don't think I can do anything about it. I loved to dance, and now, I don't trust my own feet. I loved to go to parties, but now I can't think of anything to say. I don't think it matters anyway, because no one listens to me. Work doesn't believe in me; all I am doing is putting data in. My kids don't listen to me; I don't even know why I waste my breath. The only place I want to go is my childhood home. My parents at least listen to what I say.

I feel bad for whoever is stuck with me. I really feel for Josh and my kids. I am boring to be around and moody. It kills me when someone comes over to talk to me and then goes to someone else because there is nothing to say. I can't blame them though, because I would be bored with me too.

I overheard someone say a while ago that they wished they could be me for one day. I wish I could be me too. I really miss me a lot. I dreamed of being an actress. I loved being the center of attention, and those really are dreams now. They won't come true. I am trying to have a more realistic dream now, but nothing seems to pop in my head, and I can't think of anything.

People say that "it is better to have loved and lost than never to have loved at all." I don't know if that's true. If I didn't experience life the way I did prior to getting chemotoxicity, I don't think I would miss it now. I remember how great life was, and now I dream of what life used to be. I cry because I can't experience that now. I cry because those around me have to endure the boring person I have become. I can't ask them to want to love me if I hate myself. I wish I had the courage to leave so they could live a wonderful life without me. It is not because I am trying to punish them; I truly think their life will be better without me. A lot of people go through their own hell, whether they lost a leg or were born without a chromosome.

One night, we had a party to celebrate the birthday of an amazing person. I honestly did not want to go. All that was going to happen was that I would stand there like a lump on a log and want to leave. Josh and I were going with his parents and they all really deserved to have a wonderful time. They should be able to stay as long as they want but would probably end up going home early because of me. I wished I could stay home, but then it would become a big deal. "Why aren't you going ?" "Are you okay ?" "Do you need help ?" I was tired of hearing those questions, with the eyes filled with pity that accompanied them. These are things I used to look forward to, but now I dread them.

I don't have fun anymore. I don't know why. I never understood how anyone could be so miserable. Just change your circumstances, I used to think. I knew that sometimes it wasn't easy, but it still had to be done. Now I understand. I don't think I can. Josh keeps reminding me that I should fix what I can control, my strength. He is right. It is so frustrating to have to build something back up. But I guess I need to think of it like a house of cards. If the cards fall over, even though it's frustrating to rebuild, it needs to be done.

I haven't felt beautiful since I got cancer. I don't even try to lose weight anymore or really be presentable; in my mind, it really doesn't matter. It isn't because of anyone but me. Josh, the kids, and my parents always say wonderful things to me. I think it is because I lost my confidence. I used to walk into a room and command attention. I felt great, I felt like I looked great, I spoke well, and I was fun to be around. Now I feel like when I walk into a room, I am just there. To be honest, I think we just get invited to places because Josh is a great guy to be around. He is so funny, I just laugh when I look at him. To make me laugh is no great feat, because I laugh at anything. It is hard to discipline my kids because they know it is easy to make me laugh.

Unfortunately, these days I can relate to a lot of songs. One song that I really connect with is by Justin Bieber and Ed Sheerin, *I Don't Care.* Some of the lyrics go like this:

"I'm at a party I don't wanna be at
And I don't ever wear a suit and tie
Wonderin' if I could sneak out the back
Nobody's even lookin' me in my eyes...
Don't think I fit in at this party
Everyone's got so much to say, yeah
I always feel like I'm nobody, mm
Who wants to fit in anyway?
'Cause I don't care when I'm with my baby, yeah
All the bad things disappear
And you're making me feel like maybe I am somebody.."

22

Testimony

It has been a year since my last CT scan. I should be happy as from now on, I only need to see my Oncologist yearly and get a CT scan annually. This will be my first time on this annual schedule. Prior to this, I started with seeing my oncologist every three months, then six months, then nine months, and finally, annually. Annual is where you want to be, because it is a checkup to ensure you are still healthy and cancer free. However, for some reason, driving home from my scan I had a sinking feeling, like my scan would be abnormal. Usually, I drive home just fine, but this time, I was crying. I really hope it is because my mind is playing tricks on me. My son went to the orthopedist and immediately I imagined negative things. I used to be such an optimist, but now I just think bad thoughts, and luckily it was very minor. I remember my daughter had to have a brain scan because she was having a ton of headaches. It could have been cancer, a tumor, or lack of vitamin D. I immediately thought of needing more vitamin D, which is the best case scenario, and luckily, I was right. It comes from experiences. When my family used to go to the doctor for "scary things," I would instantly think good things; now I worry about the diagnosis. Ithan just went to get an X-ray on his lower back; my first thought — cancer. Fortunately, it was nothing major, just a strain.

There is no question; such an experience messes with your psyche. I hate doctors and taking medicine. Josh always jokes that if he goes to the doctor because he doesn't feel well, they will diagnose it as cancer. I know he is trying to be funny, but underneath I believe he has a little fear. Ithan hates hospitals. Unless he really has to, he won't go.

Kobe Bryant just passed away due to a helicopter crash. It really affected me because he died along with his daughter and seven other individuals. Some people don't understand the fuss because in their minds, he was just another sports icon. He was more than that to me. I learned he granted over two hundred Make-a-Wishes. He was good with his money toward those who needed it. Unfortunately, not all famous people use their good fortune in the right way, and they eventually believe they deserve it. Also, I heard he was an amazing dad. To me, that is significant. My children are the most important people in my life. I know parents who have lost their children; I can't even imagine how they function. Kobe's wife lost her husband and daughter. We all believe we are invincible, that nothing can happen to us. I know I believed that, too. I guess the real test is how we react. I need to take my own advice. I really need to try to get out of this funk and believe in myself. I won't be like I was, which for me is a real shame, but I still can be great. I need to experience joy like I used to, smile like

I mean it, and be courageous. I used to be fearless, but now I am fearful. The Life with Cancer organization has counseling for cancer patients. I was in the mindset that if they can't make me like I used to be, why bother? But I am learning that is not true. I decided to try counseling, but it hasn't significantly helped me yet. The therapist I am seeing is nice and a great listener. She told me a great quote: "Fear is a feeling, courage is a choice." She is right. I wonder if my fear is from cancer or old age. It is probably a combination of the two. Whichever it is, I need to try to push it aside and try to overcome my fears and be more confident in myself, and as the saying goes, be courageous. It seems so easy, but when I try I get into the same funk, it just doesn't seem to work out. I need to try something different for my kids and myself, so hopefully my experience will change my trajectory. I know once I find the right path, things will start falling into place. I loved my life as it was; now I need to try and love the new me. My smile was always very obvious; I always got complimented on my smile. I believe it was because when I smiled, my whole body and soul did too.

As I am writing this book, I am reminding myself of the path we had to take. I cry as I read the posts I wrote. As tears stream down my face, I remember the pain and discomfort we experienced and I think about how our life changed, what it could have been. I have moments of self-doubt and pity. But I have to remember how lucky I am to have good friends and a great family. I quiver when I know cancer took away our savings and my ability to get a high-paying job and is one of the main reasons we are not going on vacation.

I have to remember that Iliana and I got to experience the summer together.

Sometimes you wonder what life would be like with different occurrences. We have so many. I, in particular, wonder what would have happened if my family stayed in South Africa. I definitely would not have met Josh, and Ezra would have probably not met Marla. My understanding is that when we came to America, we could have landed just outside Chicago. I definitely wouldn't have my kids, my three wonders that I can't imagine life without. I shamefully used to wonder how a parent with a special needs child could say with authority, I wouldn't want my child any other way. Fortunately or unfortunately, now I understand. I believe they mean that if their child could experience life without their physical traits that were given to them, they would be thankful. However, they are grateful for who their child is and wouldn't want them any other way. I wish Iliana didn't suffer the way she did. I wish she had what most of us refer to as a "normal" childhood. If she didn't have leukemia, who knows, she might have been this amazing softball player or gymnast, but this is the path that she was given and this was the journey that my family had to take. We could have navigated it many different ways, but this is the path we chose. Life is full of choices, expectations and determinations. It really does depend on how and which path you follow. You frequently hear of a child with a terrible childhood who decided to make their despair their reason for greatness. You also hear, unfortunately and more frequently, of a child who suffered a similar misfortune but unfortunately took a path full of corruption. Because of this unique and scary time of misfortune in our lives, Iliana is thinking of becoming an Oncologist. The money helps, but she really wants this as her career choice because she wants to help people. Sarah wants to be a child life specialist in the oncology unit so she can try to better families' lives. Who knows what they will end up doing or if something else will shape their career choices. Whatever it is, I only hope they make their choice based on their happiness and helping others.

Even though life threw a lot of scary obstacles our way, I am grateful for the many amazing people in our lives. I trust this story showed how lucky we as people can be — whether it's great friends who are supportive through life's vicious attacks, a community that shows that it will be around no matter what happens, or a loyal family who will love unconditionally through the hardest times. We are fortunate to have all three, and for this I will be forever grateful. I hope inspiration can be drawn from within the bowels of my testimony, because otherwise we will find disheartening flaws in everything. It's hard to smile through my fear of what the future holds, but I know that I will always find good in the people that surround me, and with their support, I can make confident steps toward the future too. I thank life for bringing me such goodness and am thankful for the many amazing people who inspire me.

CPSIA information can be obtained
at www.ICGtesting.com
Printed in the USA
JSHW052019050421
13301JS00003B/76

9 781946 702456